The EveryGirl's Guide® to Cooking

Simple, Delicious, Healthy . . . with a few splurges!

MARIA MENOUNOS

WITH KEVEN UNDERGARO

Z
ZINC
INK

BALLANTINE BOOKS–ZINC INK
NEW YORK

No book can replace the diagnostic expertise and medical advice of a trusted physician. Please be certain to consult with your doctor before making any decisions that affect your health, particularly if you suffer from any medical condition or have any symptom that may require treatment.

A Zinc Ink Trade Paperback Original

Photographs: Elise Sinagra

Published in the United States by Zinc Ink, an imprint of Random House, a division of Penguin Random House LLC, New York.

BALLANTINE and the HOUSE colophon are registered trademarks of Penguin Random House LLC.

ZINC INK is a trademark of David Zinczenko.

The EveryGirl's Guide is a registered trademark of EveryGirl's Guide, LLC.

Library of Congress Cataloging-in-Publication Data
Names: Menounos, Maria, author. | Undergaro, Keven, author.
Title: The everygirl's guide to cooking / Maria Menounos with Keven Undergaro.
Description: New York : Ballantine Books-Zinc Ink, 2016. | Includes index.
Identifiers: LCCN 2015048419 (print) | LCCN 2015050075 (ebook) | ISBN 9780804177146 (paperback) | ISBN 9780804177153 (ebook)
Subjects: LCSH: Cooking. | Quick and easy cooking. | Low-fat diet—Recipes. | Low-calorie diet—Recipes. | BISAC: HEALTH & FITNESS / Diets. | COOKING / Health & Healing / Weight Control. | COOKING / Health & Healing / General. | LCGFT: Cookbooks.
Classification: LCC TX714 .M4625 2016 (print) | LCC TX714 (ebook) | DDC 641.5/12—dc23
LC record available at http://lccn.loc.gov/2015048419

Printed in the United States of America on acid-free paper.

randomhousebooks.com

2 4 6 8 9 7 5 3 1

Book design by Diane Hobbing

To: Emily

BY MARIA MENOUNOS

The EveryGirl's Guide to Cooking
The EveryGirl's Guide to Diet and Fitness
The EveryGirl's Guide to Life

The
EveryGirl's
Guide® to Cooking

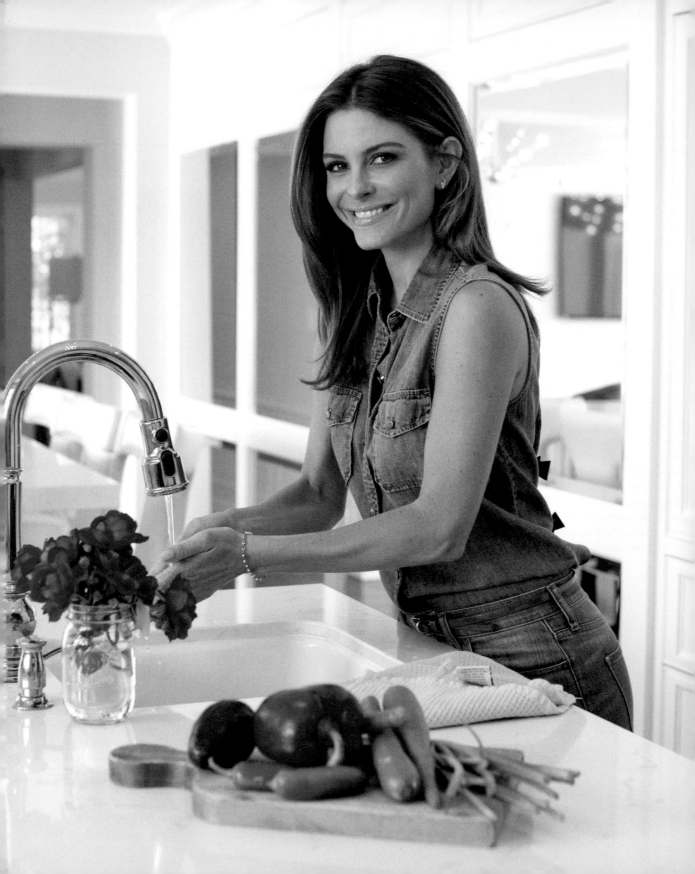

To My Fellow EveryGirls

May we—of all ages and backgrounds—continue to seek improvement, growth, and solutions in all areas of life. Let's help each other and stick together. Let's get the most out of life—in ways that are better, faster, cheaper, smarter, simpler, and healthier.

Learning how to cook for myself, and others, allowed me to finally take control of my diet. That control was one of the main factors in my 40-pound weight loss.

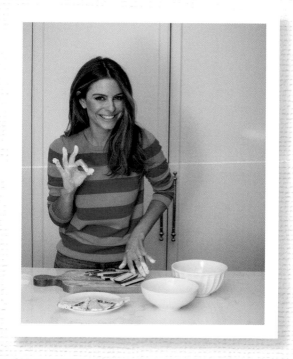

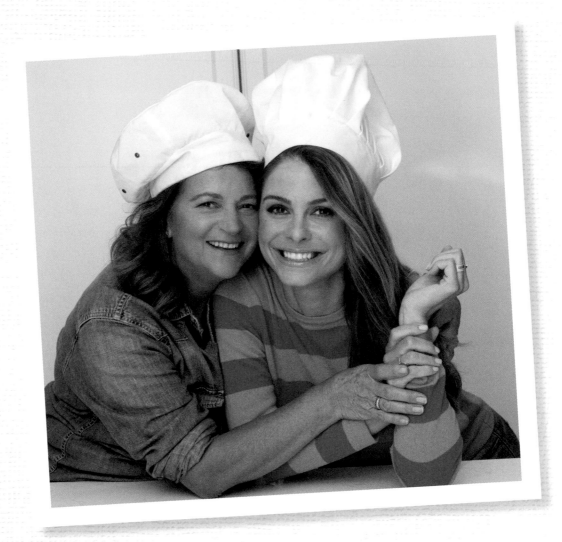

To My Mother, Litsa

By day, you cooked at the school cafeteria. Nights and weekends, you cleaned nightclubs and bars, alongside Dad. In between, you always supported my dreams—including baking for every church, school, or extracurricular event. And somehow, on a daily basis, you managed to cook the most amazing and healthy meals for the family, managing Dad's type 1 diabetes around the clock in the process. You are a culinary genius, my personal hero, and the precursor to today's EveryGirl. Dad and I are the ones in the family who get all the spotlight while you and Kev do all the dirty work behind the scenes to uplift us. And before I had Kev in my corner, I had you. When Dad fought me, out of fear, on everything from modeling, participating in pageants, studying broadcast journalism, and even my move to Hollywood, you stood by me. It was probably the only time you went against Dad, and I can't even imagine how hard it was for you to do. But you bore the brunt of it for me and for all of us. Today our family enjoys the many blessings that came as a result. You don't get nearly enough credit, praise, or thanks for everything you did for me and still do to this very day. I'm so blessed to have a mother like you and so excited to share your culinary creations with EveryGirls everywhere.

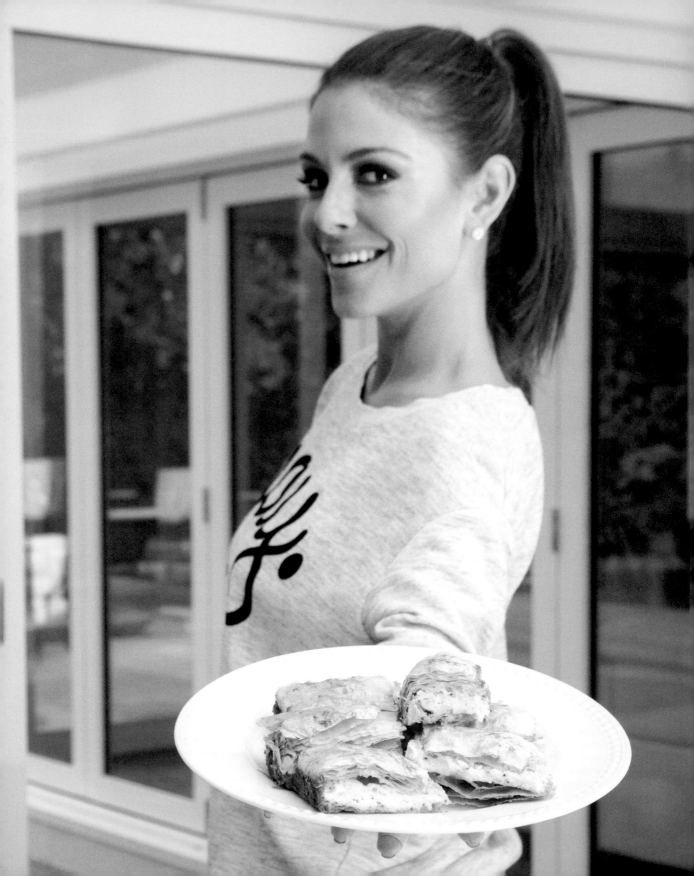

Contents

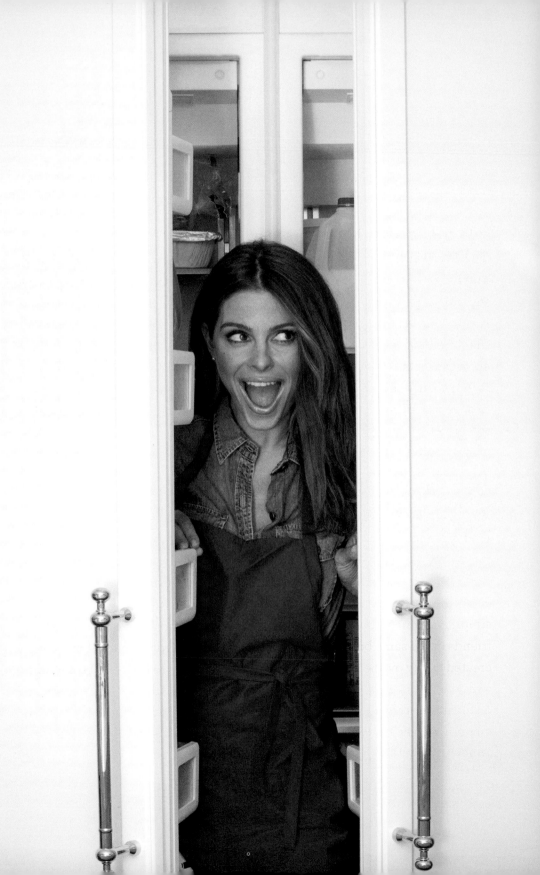

Introduction

Who Is the EveryGirl?

The EveryGirl is every girl out there who wants to try to have it all—health and happiness, and a life of meaning. She understands that if she is not growing, she is dying and that she will be learning and evolving until her last breath. She doesn't necessarily have the time and money to make it work all the time. And if she is blessed enough to have the money, that doesn't mean she needs to spend it. Whether you're my boyfriend Kev's mom, Kathie, who is in her early seventies, or one of my AfterBuzz TV hosts in their early twenties, or somewhere in between, nearly all of us can relate to the no-time, no-money, still want to grow, do, and have it all, EveryGirl predicament. And when it comes to this predicament, cooking is by no means an exception.

What Is EveryGirl Cooking?

The book you now hold is full of recipes and techniques that center on your EveryGirl needs. Whether you are experienced in the kitchen or a total newbie, this book can help you prepare delicious and healthy dishes and meals despite a busy schedule and a tight budget. My goal is to teach you how to cook unique and delicious recipes that, for the most part, are fast, healthy, simple, and uncomplicated. A few of these recipes and techniques came from friends in the same boat as me, some are ones I created myself, but most were created by my mother, Litsa. She is a woman who had to do it all—be a mother and wife, work full-time, clean, and, of course, cook. And not just cook any old dish, but ones that my father, a type 1 diabetic with extreme dietary requirements, could enjoy, too. She refused to let his dietary needs and her time and budgetary limits stop her from cooking amazing meals.

For all these reasons, her recipes, ingredients, and preparations are as simple, easy, and healthy as possible. There are no heavy creams or butters (well, except for our tiropita, see page 188), and most of the recipes keep the ingredients to a manageable number. Personally, I'm so grateful she cooks this way and that I can pass so many of her deliciously simple creations along to you. I am so disappointed when I buy a cookbook and find that the recipes include long, long lists of ingredients—including ones I've never even heard of! Likewise when the recipes require a lot of prep and experience. It makes the cooking process so daunting and discouraging, to the point I don't even want to try.

Along with keeping ingredients simple, you'll also see many similar ingredients in each recipe. This makes for a more uncomplicated shopping experience, where you're not running all over the supermarket or filling your cabinets and fridge with items you'll only use once.

So my mom can make healthy meals fast and simple. Many others can do that, too. The difference, in my humble opinion, is that Mom's meals are also delicious. I can't tell you how many people have told me, "Your mom's cooking has made me love vegetables." As you'll experience for yourself, she has a special knack for making vegetables taste incredible with just a little olive oil, some key herbs and spices, and a baking trick or two. The same friends who hated vegetables now use her recipes and make them on a regular basis.

But in all of this, I don't want health to be ignored. Some of the recipes in this book are splurge-worthy and not the most health conscious, but most do keep health in mind. I feel they need to be for all our sakes. A few months ago, I got the alarming results of a blood test that revealed I had slipped into what they term a "pre-diabetic state." Because the disease runs in my family, I have always known it could become a problem for me. The fear of developing diabetes was the main catalyst for my forty-pound weight loss years ago chronicled in my last book, *The EveryGirl's Guide to Diet and Fitness*. But today, despite a healthy weight and active lifestyle, I have to be even more careful. Now, some people might be discouraged and feel like there's no way around it, when faced with something like that. However, that's not what my mother did, that's not what I did, and it's not what the EveryGirl should do, either. Type 2 diabetes, the version I appear to be susceptible to, is largely preventable. I, for one, am determined not to get it and have adjusted my diet and lifestyle accordingly. I cut my bad carbs down, lessened my dairy intake, and focused really hard on getting my 10,000 steps in per day. But for a few months, I definitely wasn't getting my steps in, and not only did it show on my body, clearly it was reflected in my blood work too. Since making the adjustments, my current blood work has (knock on wood) shown vast improvement and I'm determined to maintain that healthy momentum.

This book will hopefully demystify the cooking process and make you more comfortable in the kitchen and in preparing your own meals. It will not only save you money, but also offer you delicious and healthy meals. It gives *you* the control over what you are consuming, which is more important today than ever; increasing rates of diabetes, gluten allergies, and countless other rising ailments are directly affected by diet. For those of you blessed to not have any ailments, don't wait for them to arise. Be proactive; take control of what you are cooking and start eating healthier. It is my hope that this book will inspire you to do that.

Your CONCERN, MY CONCERN!

Some of the recipes in this book are diabetic-friendly and/or gluten-free or can be made so with a simple swap of an ingredient or a tweak of the cooking process. Look for this icon in the pages to come. Please pay close attention to the notations that include what these swaps need to be. My endocrinologist and a registered dietician looked these recipes over and indicated which were best for diabetics and those with gluten allergies. I also included a short chapter from them later in the book explaining "good carbs vs. bad carbs" and more info on diabetic nutrition. Their names are located in that chapter as well as in the acknowledgments for your information.

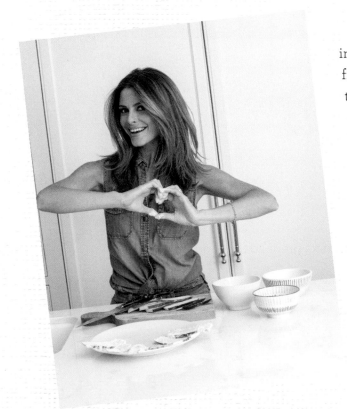

I know that some EveryGirls are a little intimidated by the kitchen. Maybe you freak out just looking at a recipe. You see the instructions and think they look too complicated, or you glance at the photo for the dish and you're positive that your version could never look that good. I want to free you of that line of thinking. Success of any kind is difficult to achieve in its own right, let alone with the mental obstacles we create for ourselves. I know there are probably other books to help women with this vital dilemma, but why not use cooking as the place to start? Loosen up and approach this as something fun. These recipes don't have to be perfect. Mine weren't when

I started (and still aren't sometimes). Also, you should feel free to interchange ingredients or portions within the recipes: More of this. A little less of that. That's what my mom and other great cooks do anyhow. Maybe that's why she and many chefs find it difficult to recite their own recipes, because they cook by taste alone! And those recipes came from trial and error and not being afraid to fail. When we experiment in anything we do, we learn. When we fail, we learn even more. As in life, failures are often our blessings. Embrace it all. Remember, if you're not growing, you're dying. Stretching your comfort level is growth; let's get growing together in the kitchen! And remember cooking is artistic, fun, and social. I love cooking with friends and I love cooking for people and seeing their reactions. My boyfriend, Kev, always had such a hard time with the fact that during holidays, on my only days off, I wanted to spend the whole day and night prepping huge meals. He'd beg me to just rest and to buy everything pre-made at the nearby supermarket! It was a nice gesture, but doing so would rob me of the best form of fun, play, and a rewarding experience.

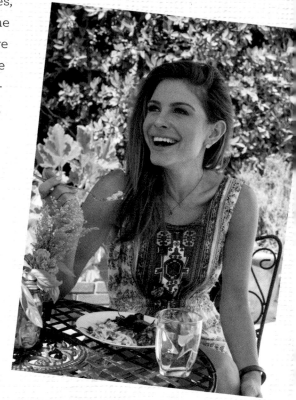

Keeping Your Mind in the State of Possibility

The long weekend in which we shot all the photos for this book turned out, ironically, to be one of the most inspirational, profound, and educational experiences of my life. However, that powerful experience, and the beautiful culinary photographs that were produced, might never have come to fruition.

Writing and creating a cookbook is far more work than just scribbling down a bunch of recipes. Recipes have to be tested, prepped for photography, and then photographed.

The "experts" that I almost hired to help produce the photography told me it would take at least three weeks to shoot the recipes. Unfortunately, with all my jobs, I didn't have three weeks. I was lucky to carve out three days! I was armed with my mom and a great group of friends who had offered to assist, but apparently that wasn't sufficient. These "experts" literally told my book agent that I was "out of my mind" for believing fifty recipes could be prepped, cooked, and photographed in such a short amount of time, and with amateurs.

I confess, hearing that had me panicked. I was crippled with stress. After all, I only had these three days to do the work and now no "expert" to produce the shoot. However, as Tony Robbins says, "stress" is just a code word for fear. At some point in the crisis, I came to the realization that my entire life, amid greater challenges, I'd been told that I was crazy and that so many things I wanted to do were not possible. I was told it wasn't possible to be an actress and a reporter. After acting in *One Tree Hill* and *Fantastic Four*, I was told it was not possible to do both serious journalism and entertainment news. After reporting for *NBC Nightly News,* the *Today* show, and *Access Hollywood,* I was told being a professional wrestler was career suicide. After wrestling on *Monday Night Raw,* grappling against one of the greatest divas in World Wrestling Entertainment (WWE) history, "the Glamazon," Beth Phoenix, I was told *Dancing with the Stars* was somehow beneath me. *Dancing with the Stars (DWTS)* profoundly affected my life, helping me form lifelong friendships and discover a passion for dancing I never knew I had. Incidentally, during the time I competed on *DWTS,* I enjoyed my life's greatest experience: wrestling at *WrestleMania* in front of 70,000-plus fans. My fellow WWE Divas and I hugged and cried after the match. Today, the WWE Divas, superstars, staff, and executives are my second family and home away from home. I'm proud of all the aforementioned feats, but I'm not writing about them to boast. The point is that when I was told that getting the photo shoot done in three days was not possible, I recalled these very memories. More often than not, I overcame the negativity of others by *keeping my mind in the state of possibility,* following my heart, and considering more what is possible rather than impossible. Whether in the kitchen or not, be sure to keep your mind in that place, too. And keep company with those who think likewise.

I remember telling the potential book shoot producer that my mom is a cook and someone who cranked out thousands of meals, daily, for school lunches. I told her my host, producer friend Tammie is a great cook herself and super creative, that my friend Susan used to be a food stylist, that my friend Marci is a workhorse who produces huge shoots at E!, that my housekeeper,

EveryGirl TIP

In running our AfterBuzz TV network, Kev swears by this motto: "Hire for heart; train for skill." In most cases, if you have heart, i.e., great passion, desire, and work ethic, you will learn the skills you need and succeed at the task at hand. Whether it's planning a baby shower, wedding, or dinner party, or just cooking in general, if you have the heart, you can make it happen.

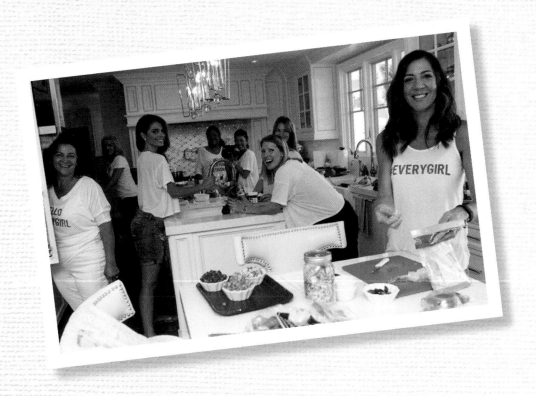

Violeta, is an outstanding cook, worker, and family member, and that my assistant, Signa, will not stop until a task gets done. Incidentally, Signa had zero cooking experience, but that was also to our benefit. She was the "canary in the coal mine," so to speak—the one to alert us of what wasn't clear and compelling to novice and aspiring cooks. To top it off, our photographer, Elise, has photographed all my EveryGirl's Guide books and pitches in to help in any area necessary. Though Susan could only help on one day, I thought, with this all-star team chipping in, the producer would surely have all the assets needed to do the job. Then I realized, upon her firmly disagreeing, that we would indeed do it ourselves. Honestly, I have total respect for what professionals are doing in this arena, but I had no choice. I also reminded myself that this was *The EveryGirl's Cookbook,* not one of those fancy chef cookbooks. It's supposed to be down-to-earth and real. Imperfections are acceptable. Thus I and my big-hearted, "can do" family and friends decided to go rogue and forge out on our own.

We assigned duties and established a rhythm, cranking our favorite tunes, singing and dancing in the kitchen throughout the process. When I spoke with the experts, I was told that shooting twelve recipes a day was "ambitious." By the end of our first day, I grabbed the list of finished recipes and started counting. 1, 2, 3 . . . 15, 16, 17 . . . 27, 28 . . . At that point, tears were running down our faces before we finished the count at 35. Everyone cheered, hugged, and high-fived. None of us had known fully what we were capable of—we just had our minds in the state of possibility. Sure, our feet hurt, but it was nothing in the face of what we had accomplished as a team. Susan was so pumped, she cleared her schedule for part of day two, but even when she wasn't there, we adapted. In less than three days, we knocked out eighty recipes—well past the fifty we had hoped for. And did I mention, we also shot the cover photo for the book? Well, we did—though doing so meant that everyone had to cook outside on the barbecue grill! Imagine, for one-third of the recipes, the ladies didn't have an actual kitchen to use—but that didn't stop them!

I was so blown away by the achievement that I had to share this story with you. I'm sure there are things you EveryGirls want to attempt in life, cooking or otherwise. I'm sure you have your share of naysayers who will say the exact

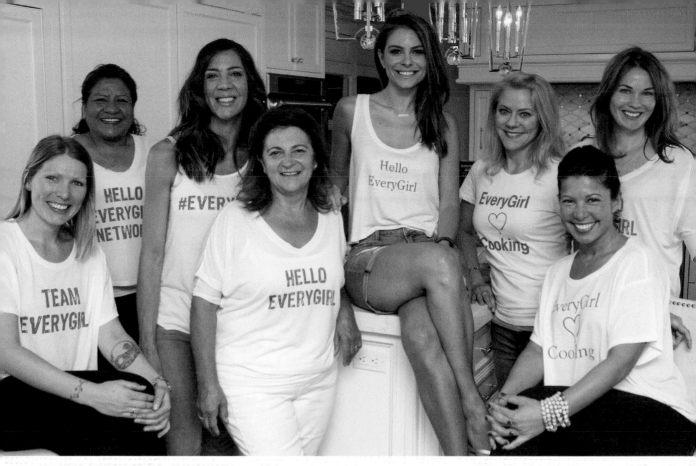

same things to you. Despite the fact I've touted the "mind in possibility" motto in each and every previous EveryGirl's Guide book, I nearly forgot it myself. That's how powerful others and their words can be—and there is no shortage of negative people out there. Sadly, most people will find ways to show you that something won't or can't work. It's just too easy not to. Surround yourself, instead, with people who will do the opposite: people who approach situations thinking about what is "possible" to achieve rather than impossible. Tony Robbins says your success is a direct reflection of the expectations of your peer group. My father, Kostas, says, "Show me who your friends are, and I'll show you who you are." My peer group is strong and I attribute much of my success to their presence. They expect more of me, think big, and sometimes even bigger than I do. Finding these people is work, too, but it's worth the effort.

Me and my EveryGirl team taking a break from our cooking to celebrate our moment! Thanks, girls, and thanks to UberPrints.com for the awesome t-shirts.

Lastly, as my dad also says, you can do anything you put your mind to. It's an overused cliché, but it's true. In life and in the kitchen, don't be afraid to think out of the box and bend the rules. Above all, keep that mind in the state of possibility.

Litsa Menounos, "Mom"

My last book, *The EveryGirl's Guide to Diet and Fitness,* was dedicated to my father, a seventy-year-old type 1 diabetic whose forty-five years of clean living and high level of activity led to proven positive results. This book, however, is dedicated to and centers on the person who prepared and fed him the most amazing and sumptuous dishes. That person is my mom, Litsa, a retired elementary and middle school cafeteria chef. The job helped to perfect her skills as a culinary artist. But, really, it gave her the health insurance benefits required to treat Dad's condition. On top of the job, she kept my father alive—literally. His constant low-blood-sugar attacks forced her to wake

Sometimes Mom and I clash in the kitchen!

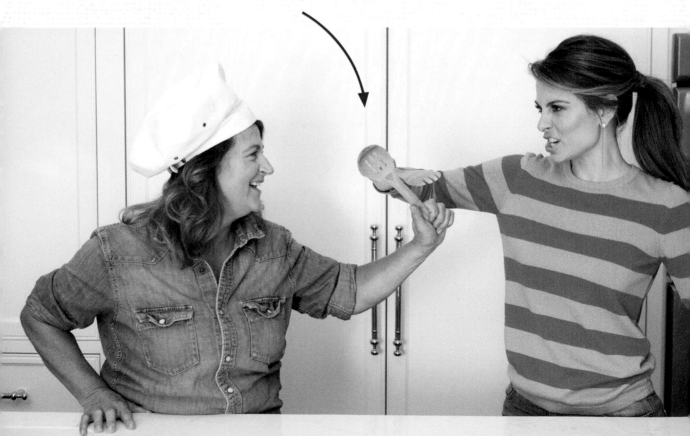

every few hours to monitor his levels and to call him on every work break to do the same. The ironic truth was, with all she had to handle, she had very little time to spend in the kitchen, yet she had to pay special attention to cooking due to Dad's disease. Her years of serving thousands of children, daily, through a cafeteria program she helped to loft from the state's lowest to highest standard, no doubt helped. In addition, my grandfather, her father, was a chef in Greece and taught her every-

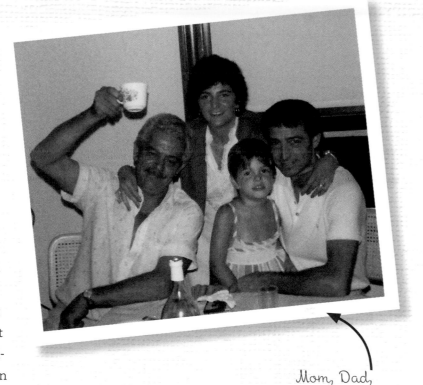

Mom, Dad, Grandpa, and me!

thing he knew. Growing up in a Greek village with little to no electricity or running water, Mom learned to farm her own fruits and vegetables—and still does so to this day. Because the family could not afford meat, they ate mostly vegetarian meals, consuming essentially nothing processed. As I wrote in my last book, I believe this diet is the healthiest around. My dad, as I constantly boast, is living proof. For all my father's impressive willpower, there is no way he would be able to be as disciplined eating-wise were it not for Mom's uncanny ability to make everything taste as downright delicious as she does. Despite everything, Mom managed to whip up the greatest and most amazing of meals on a daily and nightly basis, and I was her proud number one helper. Incredibly, she found the means to cook in bulk for all our church and family events, too, and even managed to present the food in the most stellar of ways.

The only thing I wish is that Mom's life wasn't *all* about sacrifice and family. She deserves to spend more time on herself. It's one of my personal missions to make up for things now and the reason I'm so proud to have written

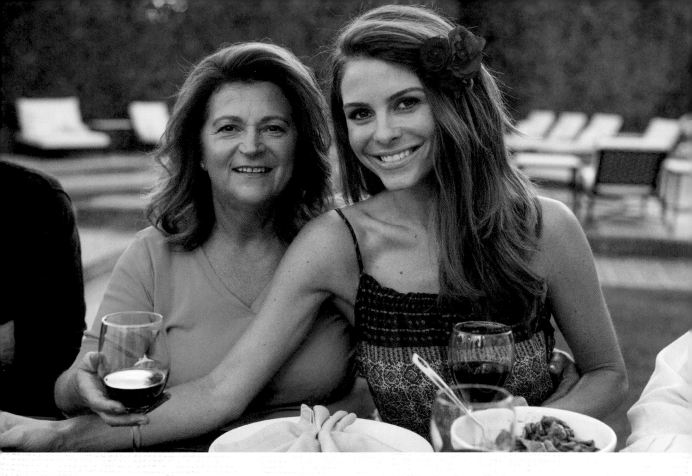

this book with her. My pride for her aside, I'm hoping that her "no time, no money, no problem," EveryGirl healthy means of cooking helps others as much as it did me. I'm hoping it helps EveryGirl out there to cook for herself, her partner, her children, her family, and her friends in a fun, efficient, and healthier way.

EveryGirl REMINDER

While Mom and I have made our best effort to create healthy meals for you in this book, not all recipes here will or should focus on health. After all, I'm a girl who loves nachos, pizza, and potato skins! It's all about maintaining balance.

As I preached in my last book, *The Everygirl's Guide to Diet and Fitness,* strive for 75 percent of your diet to be unprocessed foods that mainly "come from the ground," such as fruits, legumes, and vegetables. You can play around 25 percent of the time; just remember to *control* your portions. When you have days of eating unhealthy food—as we all do—try to balance them off with a few days of clean eating. Drink hot water throughout your day. It will suppress your appetite, help keep you calm, and detoxify you. Hydrating in general throughout the day is great for your skin and good health overall.

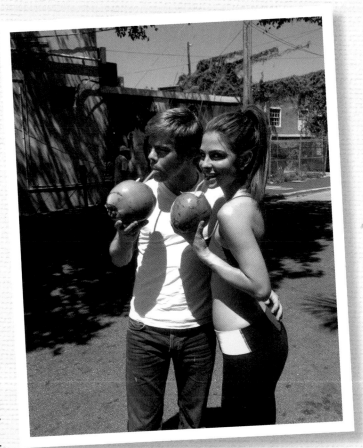

Derek Hough and I keeping hydrated, enjoying some fresh coconut water during **Dancing with the Stars** rehearsals.

EveryGirl COOKING MOMENT

English was not my first language; Greek was. That made starting school stressful and scary, but I remember how kind and thoughtful my teachers were. I also remember my sense of frustration when I couldn't understand or communicate with them. I desperately wanted to somehow connect with my teachers—even show them how grateful I was. Ironically, what helped break the ice was *cooking*! I knew a bit from watching my mom and from being her little assistant. Eggs and Cream of Wheat were my favorite dishes to make. Bringing my teachers food that I made was the only means. They seemed to get a kick out of me wanting to cook for them, but I think they appreciated what I was trying to do.

By second grade, I had a handle on the English language. Today, I have a job that requires proper speech and diction—crucial skills these teachers helped me to acquire. I'm forever grateful for their patience and care, with a nod to the art of cooking!

Hugging my grandma at my family birthday party. I was glued to her at all times. This is my favorite picture of her.

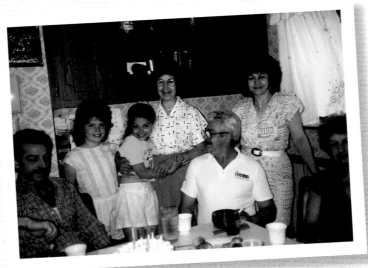

The
EveryGirl's
Guide® to Cooking

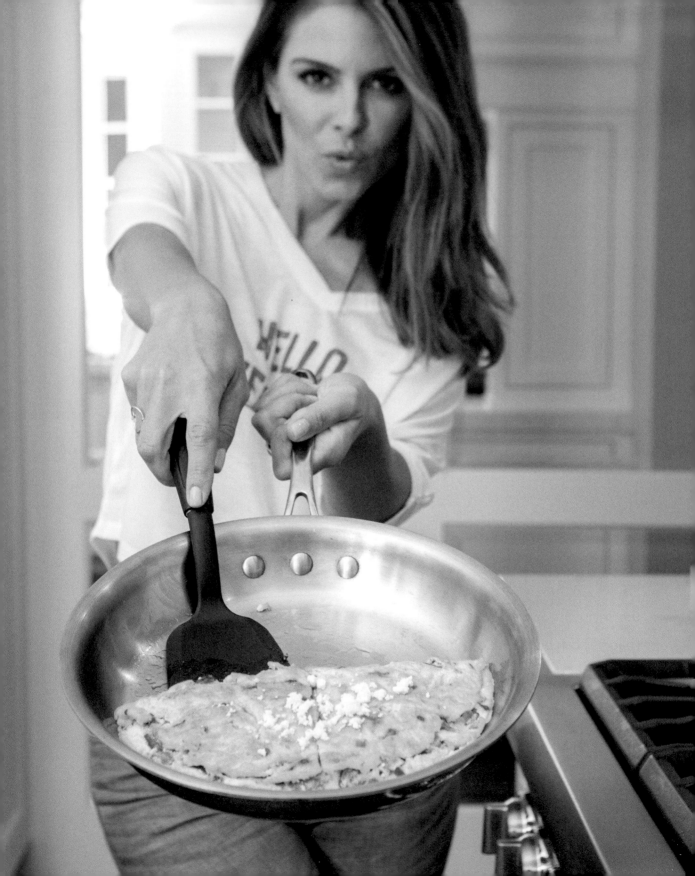

EveryGirl

COOKS BREAKFAST

Like many of you, most mornings I'm rushing out the door to go to work. For that reason, I generally like to keep breakfast simple and nourishing. However, there are other mornings, especially Saturdays and Sundays, when I like to have some fun. Whether you're heading out for a morning meeting, powering up for an early workout, or treating your family to Sunday brunch, one of these recipes is sure to help you start the day right.

Now if you feel you don't have time to make breakfast for yourself, you can do what I do: precook and prep the night before. I make a week's worth of eggs and store them in the fridge. For smoothies, I'll buy frozen fruit or freeze fresh fruit such as bananas. Many of the recipes like the quinoa breakfasts and the Banana-Ricotta Mash (page 9) can be made the night before, sealed, and stored in the fridge. They'll be there for you to consume in the morning or to grab and go when rushing out the door. Hopefully, I've left you with no excuse to have the most healthy and/or delicious breakfast! Enjoy!

Cinnamon Swirl Oatmeal

SERVES 1

For this recipe, you can use either old-fashioned or quick oats; there is no nutritional difference. However, because quick oats have been pressed to make them thinner (and thus more quickly cooked), they usually cook up into a mushier texture. As for the cream cheese "frosting"? That's just for fun! This breakfast is delicious with or without it!

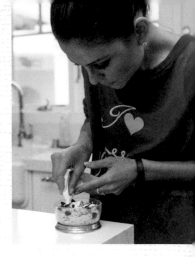

EveryGirl
TIP: I like to pre-chop walnuts or almonds and keep them in my pantry, because the last thing I want to be doing in the morning is chopping nuts! If you want to splurge, you can buy them pre-chopped.

½ cup quick-cooking or old-fashioned oats

¼ cup raisins

½ teaspoon cinnamon

1 tablespoon chopped almonds or walnuts

1 tablespoon whipped cream cheese, at room temperature

2 teaspoons milk (any kind)

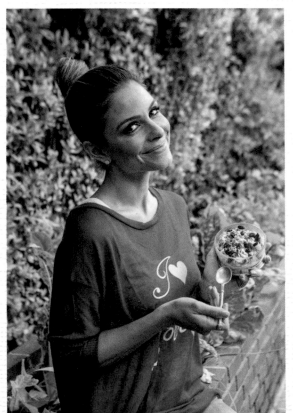

1. Cook the oats according to the package directions. Transfer to a serving bowl and stir in the raisins. Sprinkle with the cinnamon and the almonds.

2. In a small bowl, beat the cream cheese and the milk to reach a glaze consistency. Spoon over the hot oatmeal.

Steel-Cut Oatmeal with Dates and Walnuts

SERVES 2

This recipe becomes diabetic-friendly **D** if you decrease the number of dates to two.

Steel-cut oats are made from whole oat groats that are chopped into small chunks during processing. They cook up into a thick, earthy, porridge-like bowl of creamy goodness.

1 cup steel-cut oats
½ teaspoon cinnamon
1 teaspoon vanilla extract
Pinch of salt
4 dates, pitted and chopped
½ cup chopped walnuts
Milk, for serving

1. Bring 3½ cups of water to a boil in a small saucepan over high heat. Stir in the oats, cinnamon, vanilla, and salt, reduce the heat to medium-low, and bring to a low simmer.

2. Simmer for 20 to 30 minutes, until the oats are of the desired creaminess, stirring occasionally and scraping the bottom of the pan.

3. Transfer to serving bowls and top with the dates, nuts, and a splash of milk.

EveryGirl
TIP: Don't rush the cooking on this one! You want the oats to cook at a very low simmer, with just a few bubbles on the surface.

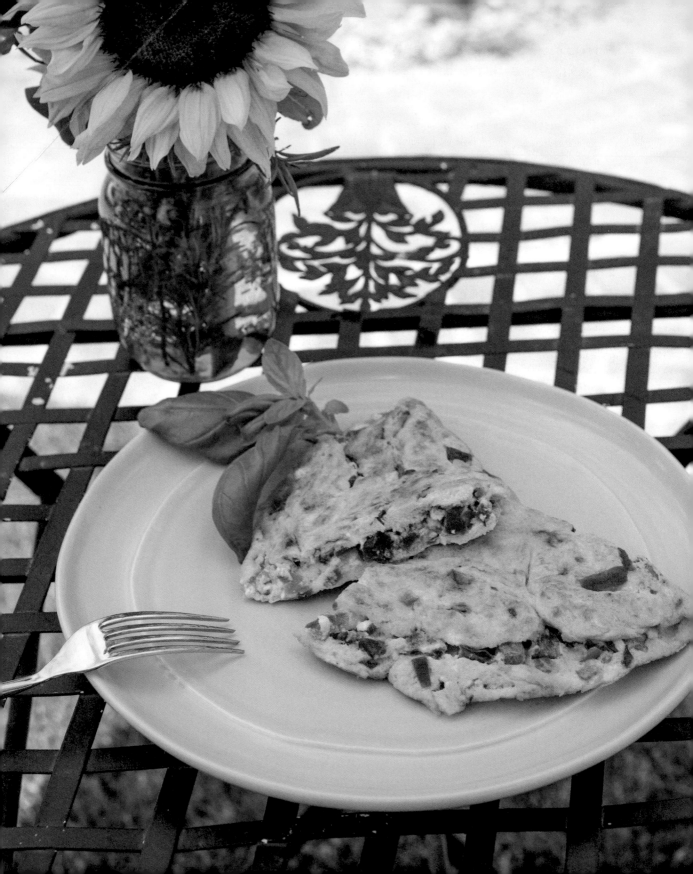

Kayiana—Special Greek Omelet

SERVES 2   This recipe is diabetic-friendly *and* gluten-free!

The pepper makes this a spicy dish. Not in the mood? Throw in some chopped black olives instead. And whatever you add, this works as a dinner dish, too. It's delicious and full of protein.

  2 tablespoons olive oil
  1 small tomato, thinly sliced/chopped
  3 large eggs
  2 tablespoons seeded and chopped serrano or jalapeño pepper, as
    desired
  ¼ cup (2 ounces) crumbled feta cheese
  2 tablespoons chopped fresh basil
  Salt and black pepper

1. Warm the oil in an 8-inch nonstick skillet over medium heat. Add the tomato and cook for 8 minutes, or until the tomato juices evaporate.

2. In a small bowl, whisk the eggs, chopped pepper, cheese, and basil, and season with salt and black pepper.

3. Pour the eggs over the tomato; do not stir. Cook for 3 minutes, or until the edges are set. Tilt the pan and let the uncooked egg run underneath the omelet. Continue this process until the top is no longer runny.

4. Run a spatula around the edges of the pan to loosen the omelet from the skillet. Tilt the pan; use a spatula to pull up half of the omelet and fold in half. Slide the omelet onto a plate.

EveryGirl
TIP: A good nonstick skillet is the key to easy omelet making. Another key? Make sure the pan is hot before adding the eggs.

Spinach and Egg Wrap

SERVES 1

This recipe is diabetic-friendly and if you use a gluten-free wrap, it becomes gluten-free as well.

When I was trying to lose weight, I made this with just egg whites and added Tabasco sauce to kick up both my metabolism and the flavor. I like spinach and tomatoes with my eggs, but you can use any veggies you like.

2 teaspoons olive oil

2 large eggs

Salt and black pepper

Big handful baby spinach

2 slices tomato

1 wrap (whole-grain or gluten-free)

1. Warm the oil in an 8-inch nonstick skillet over medium heat. In a small bowl, whisk together the eggs and salt and pepper to taste, until frothy. Add the eggs to the hot pan; tilt the pan to spread the eggs. Cook for 1 minute, or until the top is just set.

2. Run a spatula around the edges of the pan to loosen the omelet from the pan. Sprinkle the spinach and place the tomato slices over half the omelet. Cook for 1 minute, to wilt the spinach and warm through.

3. Tilt the pan; use the spatula to pull up one edge of the omelet and fold in half. Slide the omelet onto the wrap; roll up.

EveryGirl

TIP: Every time you cook eggs, the *very first* thing to do is get the pan hot. This makes for a super-quick meal and an easy-to-clean pan.

Banana-Ricotta Mash

I didn't think I would like this recipe because I'm not a big ricotta fan, but, boy, was I wrong!

½ cup part-skim ricotta

2 tablespoons sugar-free jam or honey

½ banana, sliced

4 strawberries, sliced

1. In a bowl, stir the ricotta and jam until blended.

2. Top with the banana slices and strawberries.

EveryGirl
TIP: Substitute the strawberries with any berry of your choice.

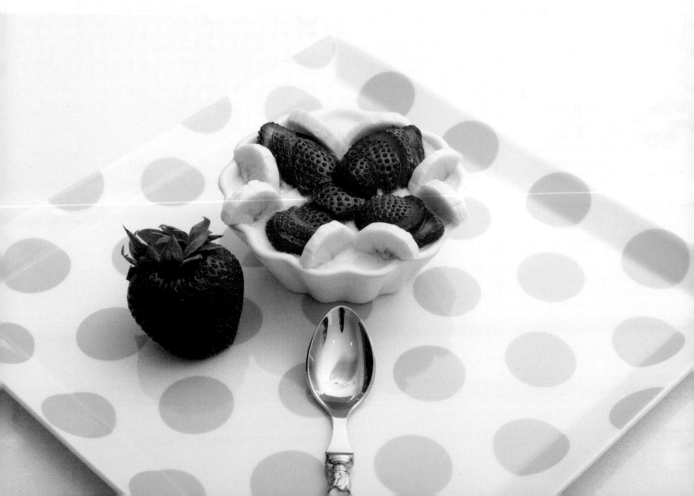

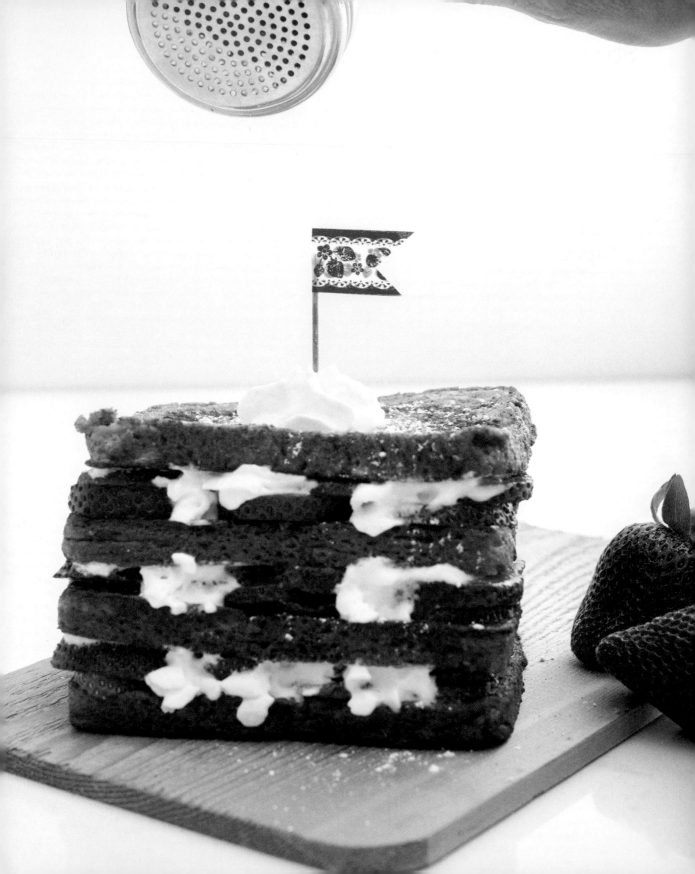

Strawberry Shortcake French Toast

SERVES 2

This is my mom's French toast recipe. She presents these pretty stacks of toast, whipped cream, and sugared strawberries like dessert—spectacular!—and, in fact, you can serve them that way, too. The whole grain bread makes it a bit less sinful.

3 large eggs

½ cup nonfat milk

1 teaspoon cinnamon

4 slices multigrain or gluten-free bread

1½ tablespoons unsalted butter

1 cup strawberries, thinly sliced

½ cup heavy cream, whipped

Powdered sugar, for garnish

EveryGirl
TIP: Don't want to bother with whipping heavy cream? Just use whipped cream from a bottle!

1. In a large bowl, whisk the eggs, milk, and cinnamon. Dip each bread slice in the mixture to coat and transfer to a wire rack.

2. Melt the butter in a large skillet over medium heat. Cook the slices for 3 minutes per side, or until golden.

3. Pile the strawberries on top of two slices of the bread; top the strawberries with the whipped cream, then another toast slice. Sprinkle the stacks with powdered sugar.

Fruity Granola Cocktail

SERVES 1   If you use sugar-free granola, this is a diabetic-friendly recipe.

This is a healthy way to start the day. Remember, however, that granola is full of both fiber and calories! A tablespoon of granola will be enough for the needed flavor and crunch.

¼ cup raspberries

¼ cup blueberries

¼ cup sliced strawberries

¼ cup plain nonfat Greek yogurt

1 tablespoon granola

Spoon the fruit into a bowl, and top with the yogurt and granola.

EveryGirl

TIP: Serve this colorful mix of fruit and yogurt in fancy wineglasses and you'll have individual portions of a healthy dessert at your next dinner party!

Apple–Peanut Butter Bites

SERVES 1 This is a diabetic friendly and gluten-free recipe!

It's kind of crazy how good a simple ingredient combination can be. Apple, cinnamon, and peanut butter make the perfect trio. This recipe calls for a healthy dose of cinnamon (which is anti-inflammatory), so be sure to use a large apple.

1 large apple, sliced

1 tablespoon cinnamon

2 tablespoons crunchy peanut butter (feel free to replace with almond butter, and for that crunch, add some chopped almonds to the mix)

1. In a shallow bowl, toss the apple slices with the cinnamon. Arrange the slices around the edges of the bowl.

2. Scoop the peanut butter into the center of the bowl.

3. When ready to eat, just dip the slices in the peanut butter. I pop these in Tupperware and eat them when I'm sitting in traffic! Keep some napkins handy, as it can get messy!

EveryGirl
TIP: Coring the apple before slicing makes the process all-around easier. You can buy an apple corer in the kitchen tool aisle at almost any grocery store. I swear by mine!

My breakfast went to Boston this morning! Ha-ha! My friend Elise, who took the photographs in this book, also took this beautiful shot from the roof of the Liberty Hotel in Boston and put it on a canvas for me as a gift. Thought it would be fun to make my breakfast in Boston.

Ricotta-Blueberry Swirl

SERVES 1   If you leave out the honey and agave, this is a diabetic-friendly recipe. It is also already gluten-free!

If you don't have any jam in the house, use honey or agave. And you can always use your favorite berries or swap in the nut of your choice.

½ cup part-skim ricotta
1 tablespoon sugar-free jam
¼ cup blueberries
2 tablespoons chopped walnuts

1. In a small bowl, mix the ricotta and jam.

2. Top with the berries and nuts.

EveryGirl
TIP: If you like this, make extra and keep in the fridge for tomorrow's breakfast! And here again, this one also doubles as a yummy low-calorie dessert!

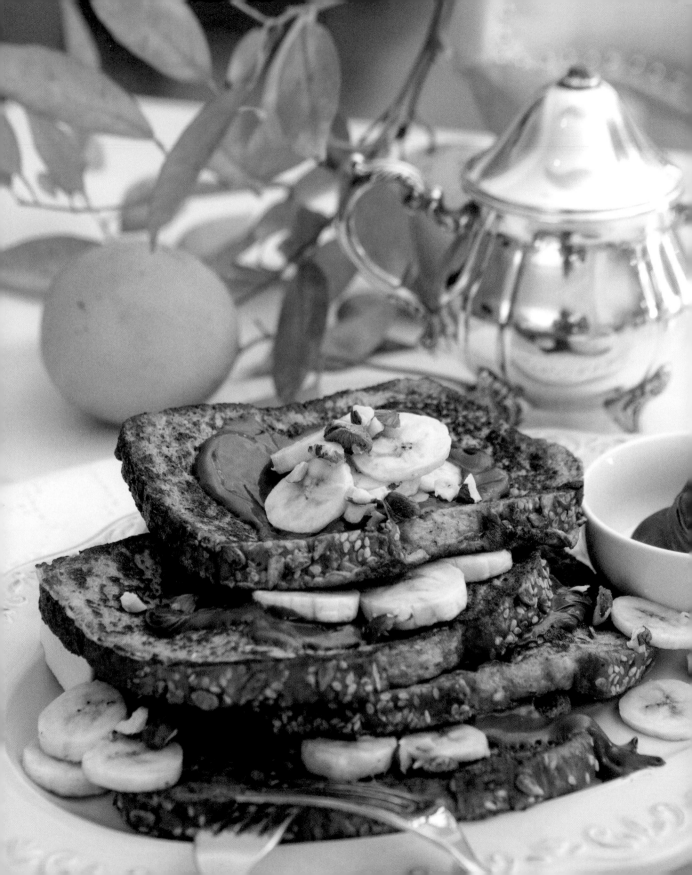

Banana-Nutella French Toast

SERVES 2

Here's another breakfast idea that could serve as dessert later in the day as well.

3 large eggs

½ cup nonfat milk

1 teaspoon cinnamon

4 slices multigrain or gluten-free bread

1½ tablespoons unsalted butter

¼ cup Nutella

1 banana, sliced

¼ cup chopped hazelnuts

EveryGirl
TIP: If you are in a hurry, skip the wire rack and place the bread directly into the pan.

1. In a large bowl, whisk the eggs, milk, and cinnamon. Dip each bread slice in the mixture to coat and transfer to a wire rack or plate.

2. Melt the butter in a large skillet over medium heat. Cook the slices for 3 minutes per side, or until golden.

3. Top each slice with 1 tablespoon of the Nutella in the last minute of cooking, to soften. Remove and stack on a plate.

4. Serve topped with the sliced banana and the hazelnuts.

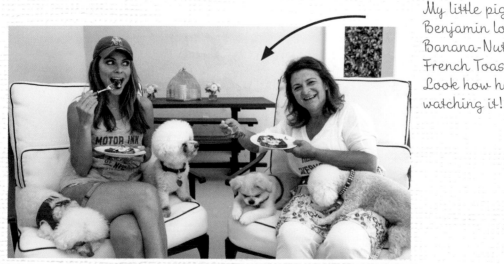

My little pig Benjamin loves the Banana-Nutella French Toast, too! Look how he's watching it!

Caramelized Onion Omelet

SERVES 1   This is a diabetic-friendly and gluten-free recipe! **D** **GF**

Caramelized onions add a deep, sweet flavor to anything they touch, but in an omelet, their specialness really shines through. The trick to getting them to that melt-in-your-mouth texture is to cook them low and slow.

    2 tablespoons olive oil
    1 large yellow or white onion, thinly sliced (julienned)
    2 large eggs (or 4 egg whites)
    Salt and black pepper

1. Warm the oil in an 8-inch nonstick skillet over low heat. Cook the onion for 15 minutes, or until golden brown, stirring often.

2. In a small bowl, whisk the eggs and salt and pepper to taste. Pour over the onion in the pan; stir to evenly distribute. Cook the mixture for 3 minutes, or until the top is just firm.

3. Run a spatula around the edges of the pan to loosen the omelet from the pan. Tilt the pan; use a spatula to pull up one edge of the omelet and fold in half. Slide the omelet onto a plate.

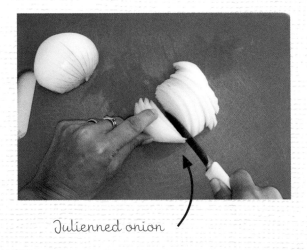

Julienned onion

Bell Pepper Breakfast Pita Melt

SERVES 1 Use a whole-wheat pita and this recipe becomes diabetic-friendly!

Pita bread is the perfect vehicle for this warm and cheesy breakfast on the go!

1 tablespoon olive oil

1 small red or green bell pepper, thinly sliced

1 clove garlic, minced

2 large eggs

Salt and black pepper

¼ cup shredded Cheddar cheese

1 whole-wheat or white pita, warmed

1. Warm the oil in an 8-inch skillet over medium-low heat. Add the sliced bell pepper and the garlic; cook for 5 minutes, stirring.

2. In a small bowl, whisk the eggs with salt and pepper to taste. Pour over the vegetables in the pan; cook for 1 minute, stirring. Sprinkle the eggs with the cheese; cook just until the cheese melts.

3. Scoop the mixture into the pita.

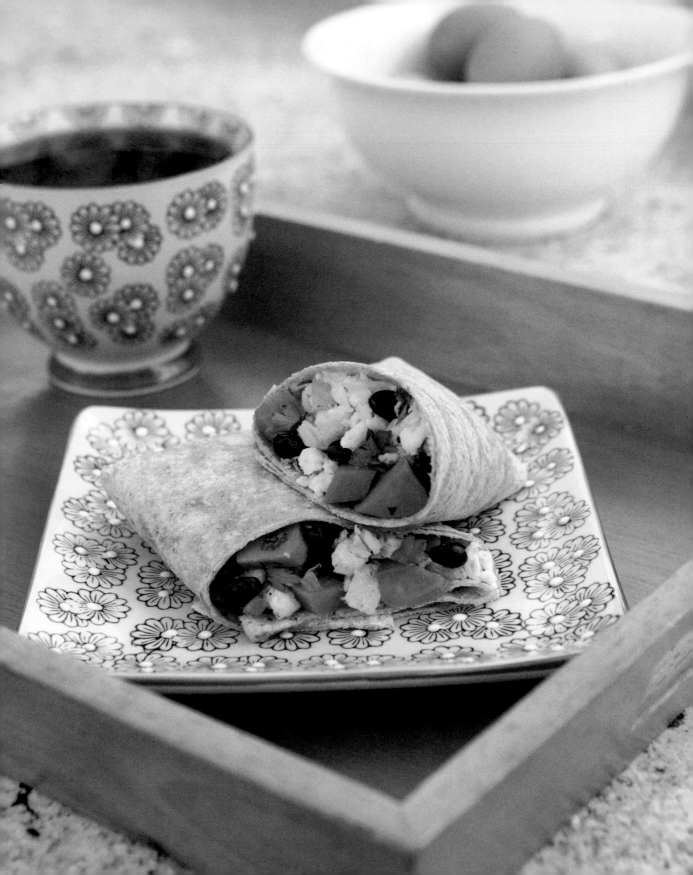

Sweet Potato and Black Bean Breakfast Burrito

SERVES 1   If you use a whole-wheat tortilla (one with less than 30 grams of carbohydrates), this recipe will be diabetic-friendly. And if you use a gluten-free wrap, it's gluten-free!

Sweet potatoes are one of the most nutritious foods on the planet, including tons of fiber in the skin. Save time and get that fiber: Don't peel the skin!

1 tablespoon plus 1 teaspoon olive oil

½ medium sweet potato, diced

½ small onion, diced

½ cup drained canned black beans

¼ teaspoon ground cumin

¼ teaspoon crushed red pepper flakes, or black pepper to taste

Salt

2 tablespoons fresh lime juice (from 1 lime)

2 tablespoons chopped fresh parsley

4 egg whites or 2 whole eggs

1 flour tortilla (whole-grain or gluten-free), warmed

1. Warm 1 tablespoon of the oil in an 8-inch nonstick skillet over medium heat. Cook the sweet potato and onion for 8 minutes, stirring often.

2. Stir in the beans, cumin, pepper flakes, or black pepper to taste, and season with salt to taste; cook for 1 minute. Stir in the lime juice and parsley.

3. Wipe out the skillet with a paper towel; add the remaining 1 teaspoon oil and set over medium heat. In a small bowl, whisk the egg whites (or eggs) until frothy. Add to the hot pan; scramble to the desired doneness.

4. Scrape the eggs onto the warm tortilla; top with the bean mixture. Wrap the tortilla around the filling.

EveryGirl
TIP: You can pre-cook your sweet potatoes and keep them in the fridge until you need to warm them up. I like this because if you want a snack in the afternoon, they are right there waiting for you.

Ruby Red Grapefruit Breakfast Blast

SERVES 1

EveryGirl

TIP: While it's good to eat grapefruit first thing in the morning (they are a good morning fat burner), this dish also serves as a delicious and healthy dessert alternative. It looks impressive at a dinner party and people love when they taste it and don't feel any guilt!

Ruby Red grapefruit sections make a beautiful presentation, especially with white yogurt as a contrast. But the Ruby Red has other benefits: It has a sweeter flavor than its yellow cousin and it also contains more vitamin A.

1 Ruby Red grapefruit, cut into sections

1 big spoonful plain nonfat Greek yogurt

1 tablespoon pomegranate seeds or a few raspberries

1 tablespoon unsweetened or sweetened coconut flakes

1 tablespoon pistachio nuts, chopped

1. Place the grapefruit sections in a small bowl.

2. Drop a dollop of yogurt over the grapefruit.

3. Garnish with the pomegranate seeds, coconut, and pistachios.

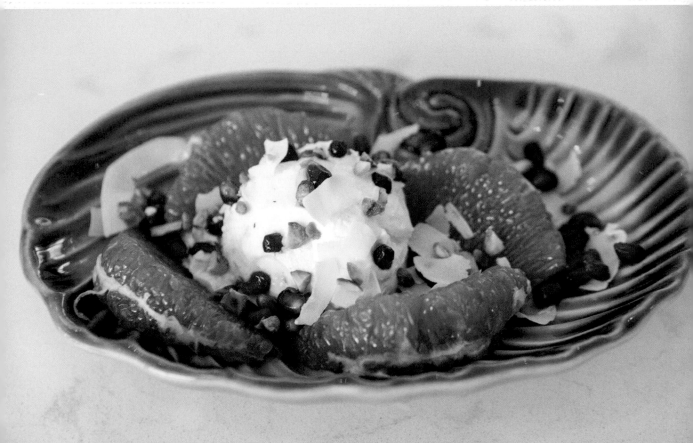

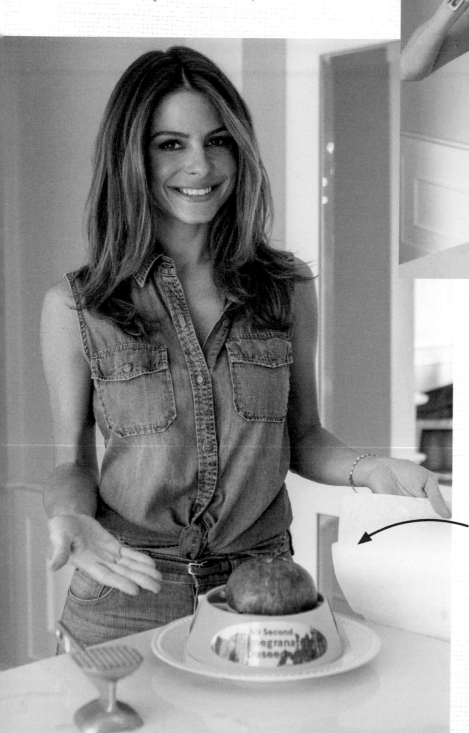

When she first suggested this recipe to me, I said, "Mom, I don't know about this one," but once I tasted it, I was hooked. I'm sure you will love it, too!

You can carefully pick out the seeds and pith from your pomegranate, or you can do it all at once with a handy pomegranate seeder like this.

Sunrise Turkey and Swiss Breakfast Sandwich

SERVES 1   Use a gluten-free English muffin and this recipe becomes gluten-free!

Fry your egg either over-easy or sunny-side up; either way works in this better-than-take-out sandwich.

1 teaspoon olive oil
1 large egg
1 slice Swiss or Cheddar cheese
1 slice (about 1 ounce) turkey
1 tablespoon prepared guacamole
1 whole-wheat English muffin, split and toasted
1 slice tomato
Handful of baby spinach leaves

1. Warm the oil in a small nonstick skillet over medium heat. Add the egg; fry until the white is set, but the yolk is still runny. Reduce the heat; top the egg with the cheese.

2. Warm the turkey slice in the hot pan near the egg; cover the pan for about 20 seconds, to melt the cheese.

3. Spread the guacamole over 1 muffin half. Layer with the turkey, egg and cheese, tomato, and spinach. Top with the second muffin half.

EveryGirl

TIP: If you're trying to be calorie conscious, make this an open-faced breakfast sandwich with only one of the English muffin halves. Cut the cheese and add Tabasco sauce or your choice of spicy salsa to help kick your metabolism into gear.

Mushroom and Swiss Cheese Omelet

SERVES 1   This is a diabetic-friendly and gluten-free recipe!

I love me some eggs in the morning. What I especially love about this recipe is that the mushrooms add a little extra protein, too.

    1 tablespoon olive oil
    6 white or cremini mushrooms, sliced
    1 cup baby spinach leaves
    1 clove garlic, minced
    2 large eggs or 4 egg whites
    Salt and black pepper
    ¼ cup shredded Swiss cheese

1. Warm the oil in an 8-inch skillet over medium-low heat. Add the mushrooms; cook for 5 minutes, or until softened, stirring often.

2. Stir in the spinach and garlic; cook for 2 minutes, stirring.

3. In a small bowl, whisk the eggs and salt and pepper to taste. Pour over the vegetables in the pan; tilt the pan to distribute the eggs. Cook for 3 minutes, or until the top of the eggs is just set. Sprinkle with the cheese.

4. Run a spatula around the edges of the pan to loosen the omelet from the pan. Tilt the pan; use a spatula to pull up one edge of the omelet and fold in half. Slide the omelet onto a plate.

EveryGirl
TIP: In order to assure a slide-off-the-pan omelet, make sure the pan is nonstick and the pan is hot before you add the eggs. You can use Pam cooking spray instead of olive oil. Also, you don't need to worry about using exactly 1 tablespoon of oil— eyeball it.

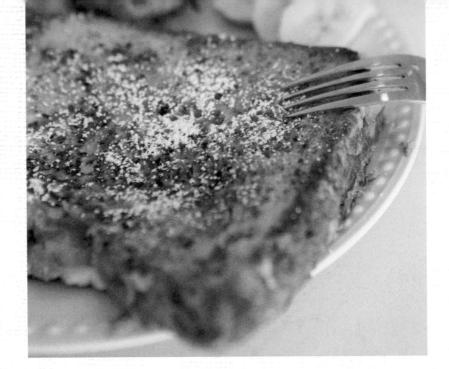

Maria's French Toast

SERVES 12

I host French toast competitions with friends. I make fresh bread with my bread maker (my obsession), slice, and then cook the thickest, most delicious French toast ever. I have yet to be beat—though a friend's French toast croissant gave me a run for my money.

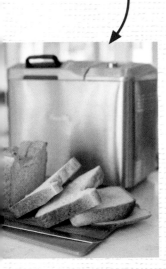

I love my breadmaker!

10 eggs

2 cups milk (any kind)

2 cups half-and-half

1 tablespoon vanilla extract

1 loaf fresh French bread, sliced thick, or Texas toast, or make your own!

Butter, for the grill or skillet (extra for finished toast, optional)

Cinnamon, as desired on top

Maple syrup, as desired on top

Powdered sugar, as desired on top

Chopped nuts, as desired on top

Fresh fruit, optional

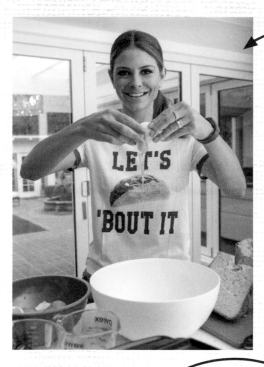

1. Break the eggs into a large bowl and beat them well. Add the milk, half-and-half, and vanilla extract, and stir.

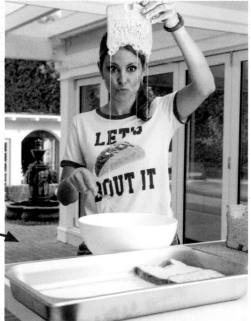

2. Place the bread in a deep pan. (The pan should be large enough to hold a big piece of bread.) Pour in the egg mixture and soak the bread in the mixture. I poke holes with a fork into the bread to allow the egg mixture to soak through. Flip if needed to ensure the mixture is on both sides of the bread.

3. Add butter to the grill or skillet, and grill the bread until golden brown.

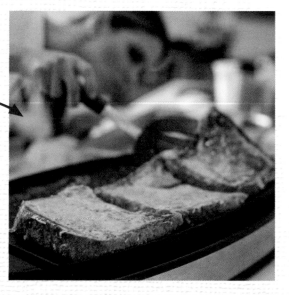

4. Serve on a platter, drizzle with maple syrup, then sprinkle cinnamon, powdered sugar, and chopped nuts on top, and dress with fresh fruit if you want.

5. Optional: For extra yumminess, add a pat of butter on top of each cooked piece.

Cheddar Fries Omelet

SERVES 2

Even if it's early morning, make sure to keep your eye on the pan the whole time; omelets cook in minutes. It's also important to use a nonstick skillet so your omelet won't stick to the pan and the pan will be easier to clean.

    2 tablespoons olive oil
    1 medium Yukon Gold or other boiling potato, diced
    1 cup baby spinach, chopped
    2 large eggs
    Salt and black pepper
    2 tablespoons shredded Cheddar cheese

1. Warm the oil in an 8-inch nonstick skillet over medium heat. Cook the potato for 8 minutes, or until browned and crisp, while stirring. Add the spinach and cook, stirring, until wilted.

2. In a small bowl, whisk the eggs with salt and pepper to taste. Pour over the vegetables in the pan, tilting the pan to evenly distribute the eggs. Cook for 3 minutes, or until the top is just set.

3. Run a spatula around the edges of the pan to loosen the omelet from the pan. Sprinkle the cheese over half the omelet. Cook for 1 minute, or until the cheese melts.

4. Tilt the pan; use a spatula to pull up one edge of the omelet and fold in half. Slide the omelet onto a plate.

Apple Pie Quinoa Porridge

SERVES 2

Oatmeal isn't the only hot breakfast cereal. Try quinoa for a protein-rich change of pace.

1 cup quinoa
2 cups milk (any kind)
1 medium tart apple, such as Honeycrisp or Gala, peeled and diced
¼ teaspoon cinnamon
Pinch of salt
½ teaspoon vanilla extract
Optional toppings: Chopped nuts, brown sugar

1. In a medium saucepan, combine all of the ingredients except the vanilla and toppings. Bring to a boil over medium-high heat; reduce the heat and simmer, uncovered, for 18 to 20 minutes, until most of the liquid is absorbed.

2. Stir in the vanilla. Transfer to serving bowls and add toppings, as desired.

Quinoa and Honeyed Yogurt Parfait

SERVES 1

This is a great recipe for EveryGirls because it's protein-packed, fast and easy to make, and great to eat on the go. You can use this basic recipe as a building block for a hundred variations. In the summer, layer in your favorite berries and top with chopped almonds. In the fall, swap maple syrup for the honey and add some chopped apple. I like it pure and simple; with just a dash of honey and lots of cinnamon.

½ cup plain nonfat Greek yogurt

1 teaspoon honey, or to taste

¼ cup chopped walnuts

½ cup cooked quinoa

¼ teaspoon ground cinnamon, or to taste

1. In a small Mason jar (or any small container with a lid), mix together the yogurt, honey, walnuts, and quinoa.

2. Top with the cinnamon.

3. Go!

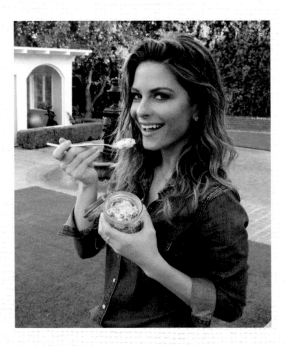

EveryGirl COOKING MOMENT

There were many days my mother would finish her job only to help my father reno-vate apartments or clean nightclubs. The two would come home exhausted and the last thing I wanted was for them to have to cook. Some of my best after-school memories are of racing home to prepare dinner. I'd make Fasolakia (green beans) or Patates Sto Fourno (oven-roasted potatoes) or other Greek dishes I had learned from Mom. It was fun and made me feel like I was contributing and helping. I lived to see their faces when they came home and saw food on the table, and got even more satisfaction when they loved it!

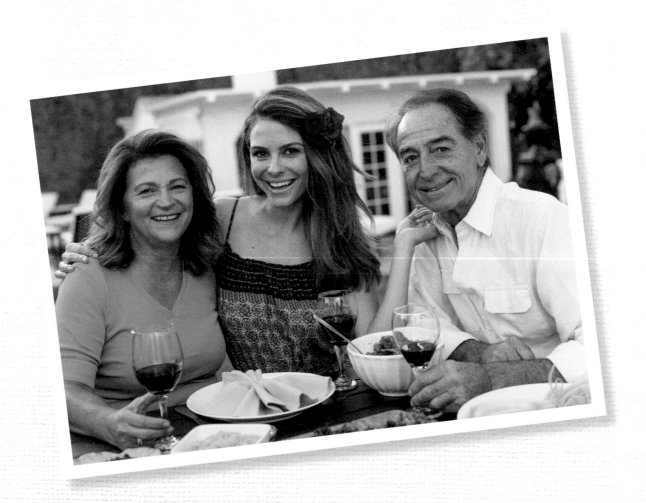

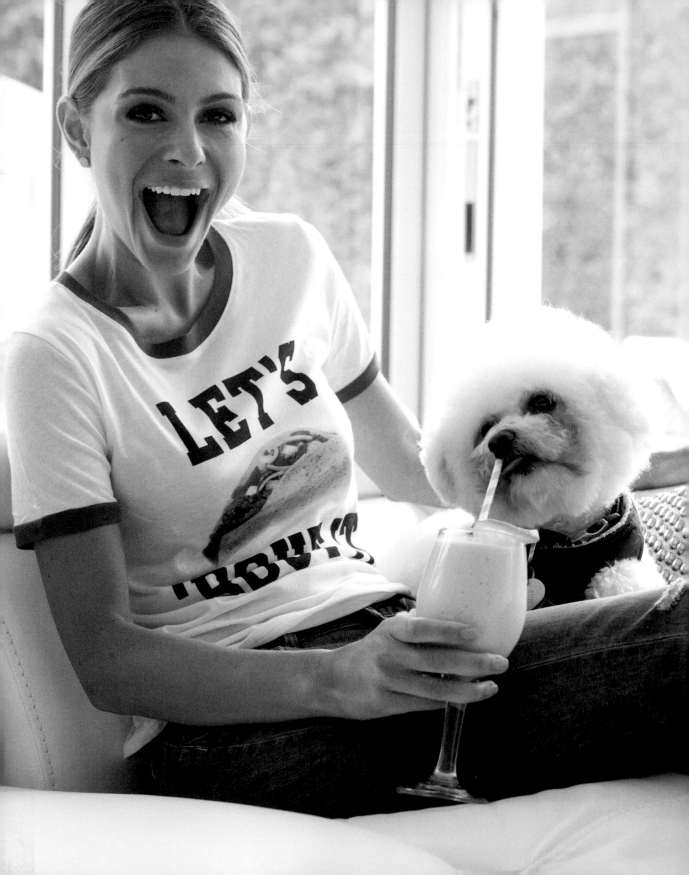

EveryGirl
SMOOTHIES

For you EveryGirls who aren't morning girls and need caffeine to start your day, I totally empathize. Sometimes we need the kind of boost only caffeine can give. My problem is that I can't drink coffee on an empty stomach. Often, I would have a healthy smoothie for breakfast, sipping it in the car, on my commute to work, then follow up with a coffee. I literally would have to lug two cups out to my car, spilling one or the other too many times to mention. . . . Want an EveryGirl solution? Try one of the caffeinated smoothie recipes in this section! Some are acquired tastes, but I'm loving them. I was careful not to add sugar and tried to keep them as pure as possible. Hope you enjoy!

Check out pages 48–50 for a few more smoothie recipes that happen to be categorized as pre- or post-workout recipes, but would be great for a morning meal as well.

Matcha Mango Smoothie

SERVES 1

Matcha powder is stone-ground green tea leaves. You can use it to make tea (no bag required!), but it's also great for smoothies. It provides a higher concentration of all the health benefits of green tea, with a great caffeine boost. For example, 1 cup of matcha tea delivers 10 times the antioxidants of 1 cup of regular green tea. I find mine on Amazon.com.

1 cup frozen mango chunks

1 banana, cut into chunks

½ cup unsweetened almond milk or orange juice

1 teaspoon matcha powder

¼ teaspoon vanilla extract

½ cup ice chips

1. In a blender or food processor, process all of the ingredients until blended.

2. Add additional ice chips to achieve the desired consistency.

EveryGirl

TIP: It's worth it to invest in a really good blender or food processor. I love my Magic Bullet!

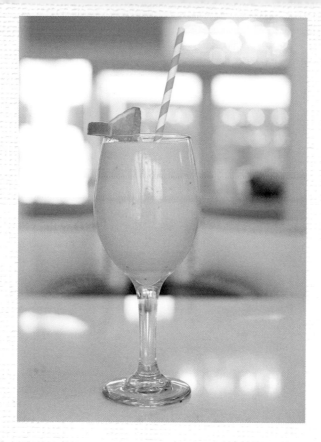

EveryGirl

TIP: You don't need to buy fresh fruit in order to make a great smoothie. Actually, frozen fruit makes for a super-cold, super-yummy smoothie!

EveryGirl

TIP: Having friends over for a pool party or BBQ? Consider spiking these delicious smoothies!

Tropical Paradise Smoothie

SERVES 2

Look at this smoothie—doesn't it make you feel like you're at a beach resort? I like that feeling whether I'm really at a resort, or at home on a rainy day.

- 1 small ripe mango, peeled and diced (or 2 cups frozen mango slices)
- 1 frozen banana, cut into chunks
- ¼ cup orange juice
- ½ cup plain nonfat Greek yogurt
- ½ cup ice chips

1. In a blender or food processor, process all of the ingredients until blended.

2. Add additional ice chips to achieve the desired consistency.

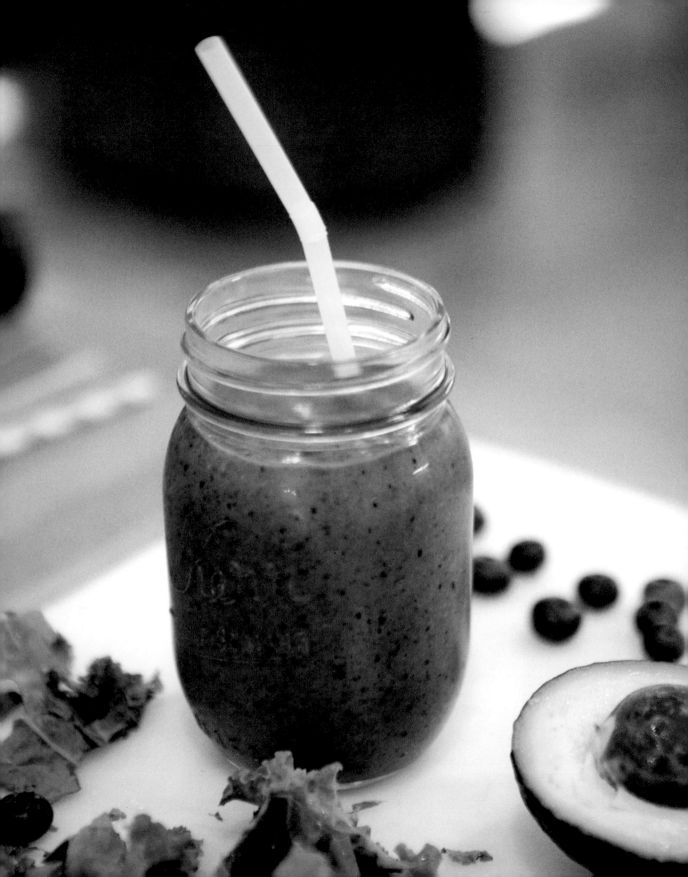

Fantastic Five Smoothie

SERVES 2

In honor of my role in the Fantastic Four *movie, here's my Fantastic Five Smoothie. I know green smoothies are all the rage, but this one will stand the test of time. It's a delicious way to get your greens!*

2 cups chopped kale

1½ cups frozen grapes

¾ cup unsweetened almond milk or regular milk

½ small cucumber, peeled, seeded, and chopped

½ cup frozen blueberries

½ small avocado or ½ small banana

½ cup ice chips

1. In a blender or food processor, process all of the ingredients until blended.

2. Add additional ice chips to achieve the desired consistency.

EveryGirl
TIP: Remember to slice off the tough inner rib of the kale—you only want to add the leaves.

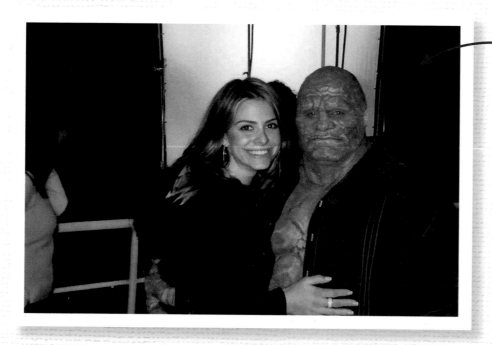

On the set of the ~~Fantastic Four~~ with "The Thing," Michael Chiklis, who is now a dear friend.

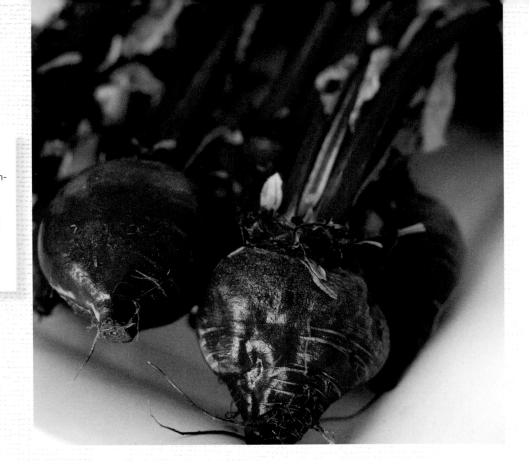

EveryGirl

TIP: Look for vacuum-packed beets in the produce section. They are already cooked and peeled and specially sealed to maintain freshness.

Sweet Beet and Berry Smoothie

SERVES 1

Not only is this smoothie pretty in color, it's also packed with antioxidants!

> 1 medium cooked and peeled beet, finely chopped
> ½ cup frozen blueberries
> ½ cup frozen strawberries
> ½ cup pomegranate juice
> ½ cup kale or Swiss chard leaves
> ½ cup ice chips

1. In a blender or food processor, process all of the ingredients until blended.

2. Add additional ice chips to achieve the desired consistency.

Coffee-Coconut-Almond Frosty

SERVES 1

Get your caffeine buzz and a healthy start all in one glass!

- ½ cup unsweetened almond milk or regular milk
- ½ cup cold coffee
- ½ frozen banana, chopped
- ½ teaspoon vanilla extract
- 1 teaspoon coconut oil
- ¼ cup unsweetened coconut flakes
- 1 cup ice chips
- Chopped almonds, for topping

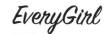

EveryGirl **TIP:** You can blend the coconut flakes into the smoothie or sprinkle them on top. Serve with a long spoon to scoop up the crunchy nuts and sweet coconut.

1. In a blender or food processor, process all of the ingredients except the almonds until blended.

2. Add additional ice chips to achieve the desired consistency. Top with the chopped almonds.

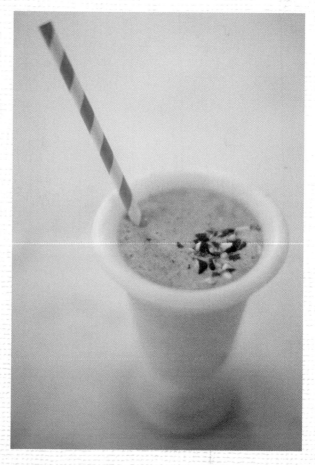

Green Java Smoothie

Add intense coffee flavor by making frozen coffee cubes for your smoothies. Whenever you have leftover coffee in the morning, pour it into an ice cube tray so you always have some in the freezer.

1 cup unsweetened almond or regular milk

5 frozen coffee cubes

½ cup baby spinach

½ cup avocado

½ cup frozen green grapes

1 tablespoon unsweetened cocoa

In a blender or food processor, process all of the ingredients until blended.

Banana-Coffee Smoothie

SERVES 1

My personal favorite!

½ cup strong coffee, cold
1 frozen banana, cut into chunks
¼ cup coconut milk or any milk
1 tablespoon ground flaxseed
½ cup ice chips
1 tablespoon sweetened or unsweetened coconut flakes

1. In a blender or food processor, process all of the ingredients except the coconut flakes until blended.

2. Add additional ice chips to achieve the desired consistency.

3. Garnish with the coconut flakes.

EveryGirl
TIP: Flaxseed delivers an extra dose of fiber and omega-3 acids to this creamy drink. But if you don't have it on hand, make the smoothie anyway!

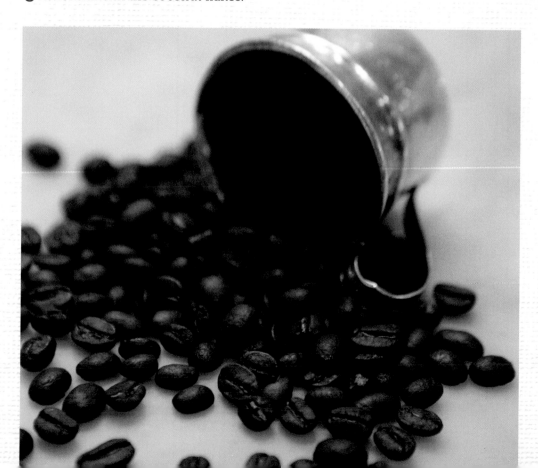

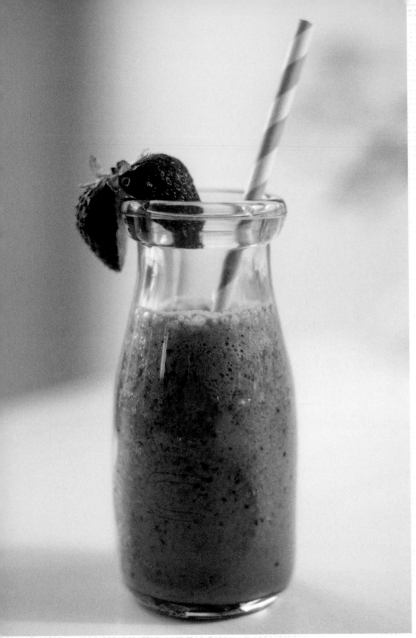

Green Tea and Berry Blast

SERVES 1

Need a healthy kick? This should do it for ya!

1 green tea bag
1 cup boiling water
1 cup frozen berries (any kind)
½ frozen banana, chopped
½ cup plain nonfat Greek yogurt
½ cup water
1 tablespoon ground flaxseed, optional

1. Add the tea bag to the boiling water and remove after 10 minutes.

2. Pour the tea into an ice cube tray and freeze.

3. In a blender or food processor, process 4 frozen tea cubes with the berries, banana, yogurt, water, and flaxseed, if using, until blended.

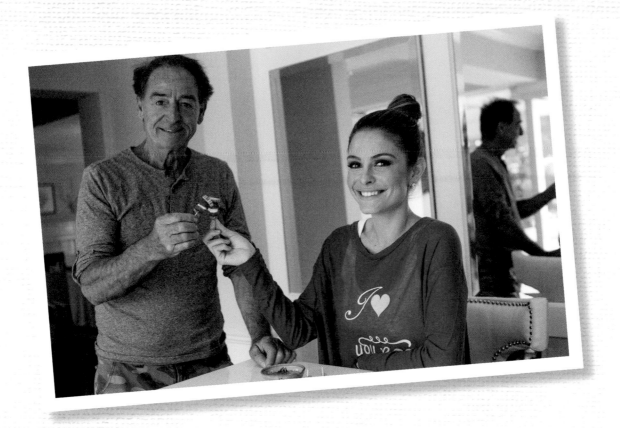

EveryGirl COOKING MOMENT

Around my dad's birthday, or Greek name day, I have always made him cakes or desserts. Since he's a diabetic who steers clear of refined sugar, creating such treats has proved challenging—but also fun. When I was young, I'd have to get innovative, like using almonds to create designs on top of the cakes. I don't know how good they were back then, but Dad never let on, either way. He loved the fact that I made the effort and always ate it all up!

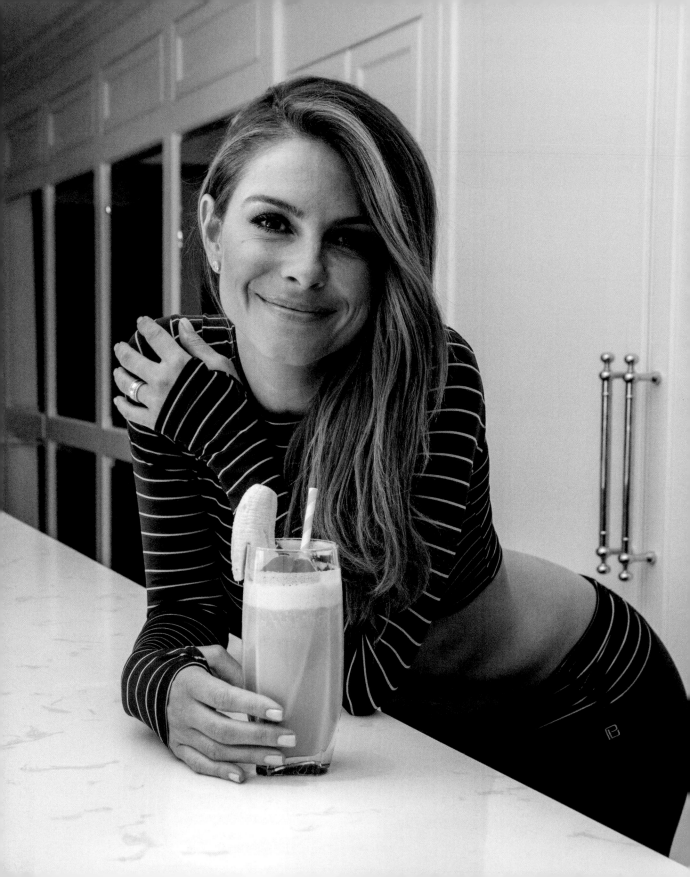

EveryGirl
WORKS OUT

If you're an early riser, you may exercise best on an empty stomach. But for many of us, a little something in our stomach helps to give us that much-needed boost to get moving. Generally, nutrition experts recommend loading up on carbs, both simple and complex, *before* working out. Simple (but healthy!) sugars provide a blast of energy (think fresh and dried fruit), while complex carbs (like oatmeal and whole-grain bread) gradually release energy throughout the workout. Post-workout, reach for protein-rich foods to help aid in muscle recovery. You'll want nutrient-dense, fiber-rich foods to fill you up, but not weigh you down. Protein shake, anyone?

Check out pages 54–56 for my protein snack ideas; many of them would be great pre- or post-workout.

Turkey, Provolone, and Lettuce Wrap

SERVES 2   This is a diabetic-friendly and gluten-free recipe!

You can use iceberg or Boston lettuce leaves in place of the romaine for this recipe, if you prefer. Just make sure the leaf is large enough to contain all these yummy ingredients.

½ ripe avocado, sliced

2 tablespoons plain nonfat Greek yogurt

Squeeze of fresh lemon juice

Salt and black pepper

4 large romaine lettuce leaves

4 slices (4 ounces) turkey

1 small tomato, thinly sliced

4 thin slices Provolone or Swiss cheese

1. In a small bowl, mash the avocado with a fork, then add the yogurt, lemon juice, and salt and pepper to taste. Mash until blended and creamy.

2. Flatten the lettuce leaves on a counter. Layer with the turkey, avocado cream, tomato, and cheese. Roll up.

Green Omelet

SERVES 1   This is a diabetic-friendly and gluten-free recipe!

I've got breakfast recipes that double as desserts, so why not a recipe made up of traditionally breakfast-time ingredients served up post-workout?

  2 tablespoons olive oil
  1 small red onion, sliced
  ½ small green pepper, sliced
  ½ small red pepper, sliced
  3 handfuls baby spinach
  1 clove garlic, minced
  4 egg whites or 2 whole eggs
  Salt and black pepper

1. Warm the oil in an 8-inch nonstick skillet over medium heat. Add the onion and the green and red peppers; cook for 3 minutes, stirring.

2. Stir in the spinach and garlic; cook for 2 minutes. Remove from the pan and set aside.

3. In a bowl, whisk the egg whites (or eggs) and salt and pepper to taste. Add to the hot pan. Cook for 3 minutes, until the top is just set.

4. Run a spatula around the edges of the pan to loosen the omelet from the pan. Sprinkle the spinach mixture over half the omelet. Cook for 1 minute, to warm through.

5. Tilt the pan; use a spatula to pull up one edge of the omelet and fold in half. Slide the omelet onto a plate.

Green Power Smoothie

SERVES 1

Smoothies are the perfect post-workout snack—everything you need to replenish your tired body and stoke its fire for the rest of the day!

1 frozen banana, cut into chunks

1 cup packed spinach or kale leaves

½ cup apple cider or apple juice

½ cup unsweetened applesauce

½ cup plain nonfat Greek yogurt

½ cup ice chips

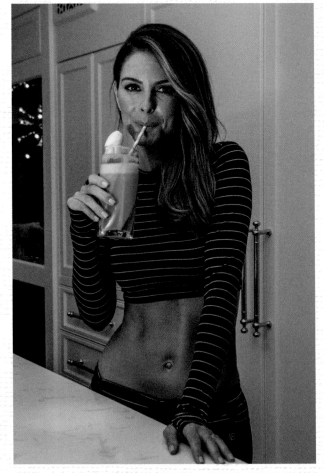

1. In a blender or food processor, process the banana, spinach or kale leaves, juice, applesauce, yogurt, and ice chips until blended.

2. Add additional ice chips to achieve the desired consistency.

EveryGirl
TIP: Either a blender or a food processor works to whip up this mean, green super-nutritious smoothie. I have a Magic Bullet and it's perfect.

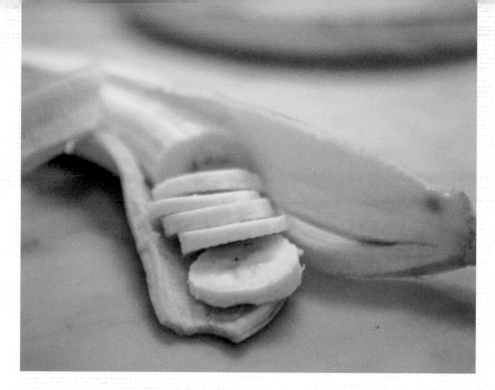

EveryGirl
TIP: The trick to a
creamy smoothie is to
blend it longer than you
think you need to.

Banana-Date Shake

SERVES 1

Use fewer dates if you want to bring down the sugar content here!

  1 frozen banana, cut into slices
  3 dates, pitted and coarsely chopped
  ½ cup plain nonfat Greek yogurt
  ¼ cup nonfat milk
  ½ cup ice chips
  ⅛ teaspoon cinnamon

1. In a blender or food processor, process all of the ingredients except the cinnamon, until blended.

2. Add additional ice chips to achieve the desired consistency.

3. Sprinkle the cinnamon over the smoothie.

Pom-Berry Blast Smoothie

SERVES 1

If you feel a little run down, this has everything you need: antioxidants and vitamin C.

1 cup frozen blueberries or strawberries, or mixed berries
½ cup plain nonfat Greek yogurt
½ cup unsweetened pomegranate juice
¼ cup orange juice
½ cup ice chips

1. In a blender or food processor, process all of the ingredients until blended.

2. Add additional ice chips to achieve the desired consistency.

EveryGirl

TIP: This is no sweet treat, but an intensely flavored, extra-nutritious morning wake-me-up. Add some honey or agave if you'd like it sweeter.

EveryGirl

TIP: In case you're wondering about the shirt, it's the online broadcast network Kev and I created that produces "after-shows" for your favorite TV shows, while helping hosts like me build their brands and careers. My mom brings food to the AfterbuzzTV studio weekly, when she's in town. She even gives cooking lessons to our hosts.

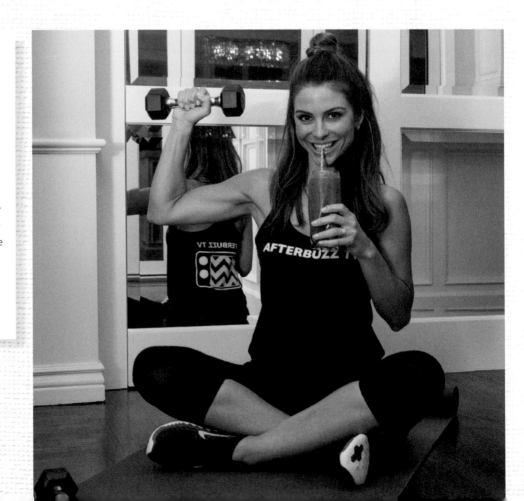

Peanut Butter Breakfast Sandwich

SERVES 1

So simple, yet so delicious. If you prefer almond butter, it's an easy swap. Also, if you don't like ricotta, try banana.

    2 slices whole-grain or gluten-free bread
    1 tablespoon sugar-free peanut butter or almond butter
    2 tablespoons part-skim ricotta cheese
    ½ small apple, thinly sliced

1. Toast the bread.

2. Spread the peanut butter on one warm bread slice, the ricotta on the other.

3. Layer the apple slices on top of the peanut butter and top with the ricotta-covered slice of bread.

EveryGirl
TIP: Serve this protein-packed sandwich pre- or post-workout, or as an afternoon snack.

Yogurt Cup Crunch

SERVES 1

Greek yogurt is thicker in texture and higher in protein than regular yogurt. Rather than buying flavored kinds, stir in your own flavors and sweeteners, like fruit and sugar-free syrup.

EveryGirl
TIP: Reduce the calories in this dish by omitting half the granola and half the nuts.

½ cup plain nonfat Greek yogurt

2 tablespoons sugar-free syrup or jam

1 small apple, diced

2 tablespoons unsalted chopped cashews or other nut

2 tablespoons granola or other high-fiber cereal

1. In a small cup, blend the yogurt and syrup.

2. Stir in the apple, cashews, and granola.

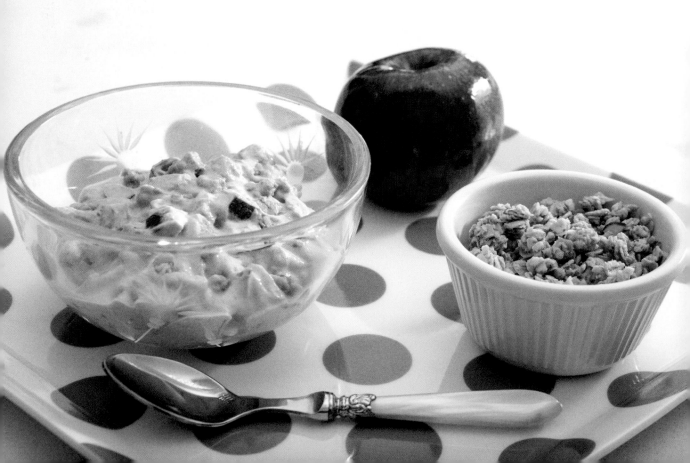

EveryGirl COOKING MOMENT

If you haven't already guessed by now, cooking is one of the easiest and finer ways of showing love and appreciation. When Kev and I first started dating, it was rough times. He isn't Greek, so my family didn't accept him, or me, because of it. On top of that, he was deep in debt over the making of his first film and I lost my college tuition to Emerson College in the process. My parents and I had such a disconnect over my dating Kev that they refused to help pay my tuition. I had loans in my name, but they weren't enough. For over a year Kev worked three jobs, seven days a week: construction by day, bartending by night, and carnival work on the weekends. Physically, it was brutal labor and involved little sleep, but he powered through. Mentally, however, it was heartbreaking. A 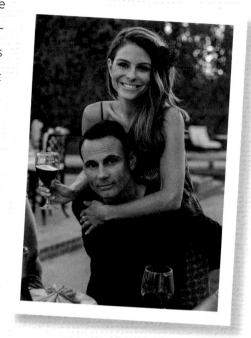 year later he was a head writer at MTV with a bright Hollywood future. Yet, he managed to pay off his debts and mine as well as my tuition for community college while supporting us both in the process. In that period, I went to Bunker Hill Community College, did his laundry, and all else I could to help him along—including making his lunches and dinners so we could save money. He always said that just having those meals to look forward to got him through. Part of it was having something delicious to enjoy, but most of it was knowing that, through those meals, he had someone in the world who loved him, stood by him, and hadn't given up on him. Another example of the vast power of cooking.

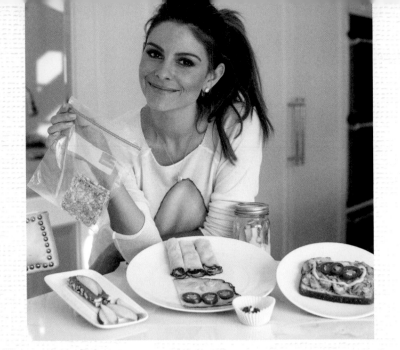

EveryGirl

TIP: Stock your fridge, your car, your desk at work, with satisfying, healthy protein snacks like almonds. They're invaluable for days when you're on the road for work, need an afternoon boost, or crave just a little something before a workout.

EveryGirl Gets Her Protein Snack

Except for the Green Baked Potato and "Buttered" Toast, these quick-fix protein snacks are all diabetic-friendly and gluten-free! **D** **GF**

EveryGirl knows that protein is one of the building blocks of a strong and healthy body. Protein provides long-lasting energy and leaves you satisfied for a long time. For me, real-food protein snacks help on days when I'm rushing and need something that will curb my hunger and steer me away from mindless munching. They can also be a great pre- and post-workout pick-me-up!

Below are some of my quick-fix, hunger-busting ideas to help you reach your recommended protein intake in easy and tasty ways.

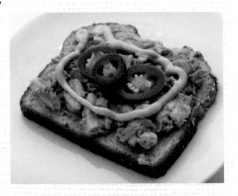

- **Spicy Avocado Toasts**—Mash half of a small avocado and spread on whole-grain (or gluten-free) toast. Top with sliced jalapeño and a squeeze of lemon juice or spicy mustard.

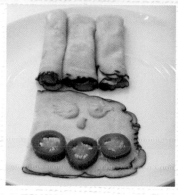

- **Turkey-Lettuce Wrap**—Spread some spicy mustard on a slice of turkey. Wrap it up in a soft leaf of butter lettuce.

- **Spicy Turkey Wrap**—Spread some spicy mustard on a slice of turkey, add a couple of sliced jalapeños, and roll into a wrap. If you're making several of them, use toothpicks to hold the wrap together.

- **Curried Bean Salad**—Mash drained canned white beans with tahini, lots of lemon juice, and some curry powder. Stir in shredded carrots and sliced scallions. Top with dried cranberries and some chopped cashews and serve on a bed of spring greens or stuffed into a whole-grain pita.

- **Protein Nut Mix**—Almonds pack more protein than most other nuts. Toss almonds with dried fruit and popcorn for extra fiber. Fill a baggie with this homemade trail mix and keep it at your desk or in your car.

- **Hummus to Go**—Spoon hummus into the bottom of a small Mason jar. Add sliced veggies (like celery sticks, raw green beans, and baby carrots), poking them into the hummus. Screw the top on the jar and head out the door!

- **Chickpea Poppers**—Note: This one has a bit of prep time, but it's a great yummy protein snack! Toss a can of drained chickpeas with olive oil, garlic powder, cumin, and salt and pepper. Roast in a 400°F oven for 30 minutes, or until dry and golden, shaking the pan occasionally.

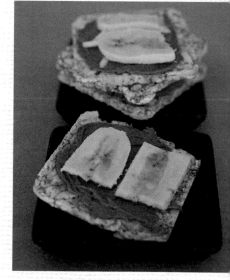

- **Almond Butter Cracker**—Spread some almond butter and sliced banana on a spelt-flaxseed cracker. Make it as a sandwich or leave as is.

- **Black Bean Salsa Wrap**—Toss drained black beans with quartered cherry tomatoes, cumin, salt, and a healthy squeeze of lime juice. Wrap in a whole-grain flour tortilla.

- **Green Baked Potato**—Potatoes and green peas have a surprising amount of protein for such unassuming veggies. Bake a russet potato in the microwave for 10 to 12 minutes, until cooked through, turning occasionally. Scoop out some of the insides of the potato and discard (or save for another use) and fill with thawed peas while the potato is still hot (to warm the peas). Top with a dollop of plain Greek yogurt and a sprinkle of chopped chives.

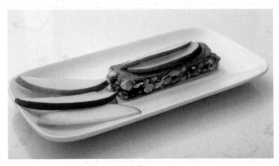

- **Speedy Egg Salad**—Smash up a hard-boiled egg with some mustard and salt. Spread on whole-grain (or gluten-free) toast or scoop up with celery sticks.
- **Apple-Almond Bar**—Spread almond butter or cashew butter on a thin protein bar. Top with sliced apples.
- **Cucumber Snack**—Thickly slice a cucumber. Top with a dollop of prepared hummus.
- **Cottage Cheese Snack**—Top cottage cheese with quartered cherry tomatoes, chopped fresh parsley, and a sprinkle of sunflower seeds.
- **"Buttered" Toast**—Spread some almond butter on whole-grain (or gluten-free) toast. Top with shredded carrots and sprouts. Don't like that? Use chopped almonds, walnuts, and flaxseed.
- **Compost Crunch**—A plain cup of cereal is a bit boring. In a baggie, mix high-fiber cereal, some spicy nut mix, and some dried fruit or goji berries.
- **Stuffed Dates**—Stuff pitted dates with low-fat cream cheese and chopped almonds.
- **DIY Popcorn**—Toss 2 cups warm plain popcorn with 2 tablespoons grated Parmesan, some garlic powder, and salt. Or toss the warm popcorn with some finely grated dark chocolate and some dried cherries.

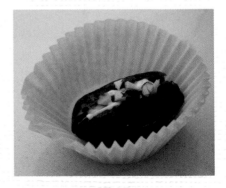

- **Balsamic Strawberries and Greek Yogurt**—Drizzle sliced strawberries with balsamic vinegar. Spoon over Greek yogurt. Sprinkle with mint if you have it.

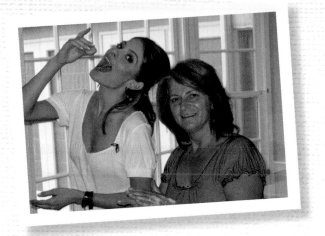

EveryGirl COOKING MOMENT

My mom and I, together and separately, have always cooked for my bosses and co-workers. I love getting our crew involved in cook-offs, where everyone brings in their "go-to" signature dish! At lunch, we all gorge on everyone's recipes, then vote to determine the best. I bring a prize for the winner. It's a fun way to build team spirit. It's also fun to cook for coworkers who may have to work holidays, are burning the candle on both ends, or just need something to brighten up their week. At *Extra,* the crew works every Christmas Eve, so Mom and I always brought over platters and trays of food, including a recipe I got at a friend's cook-off years earlier!

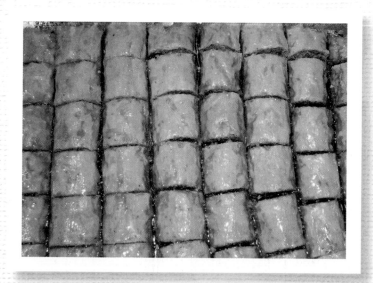

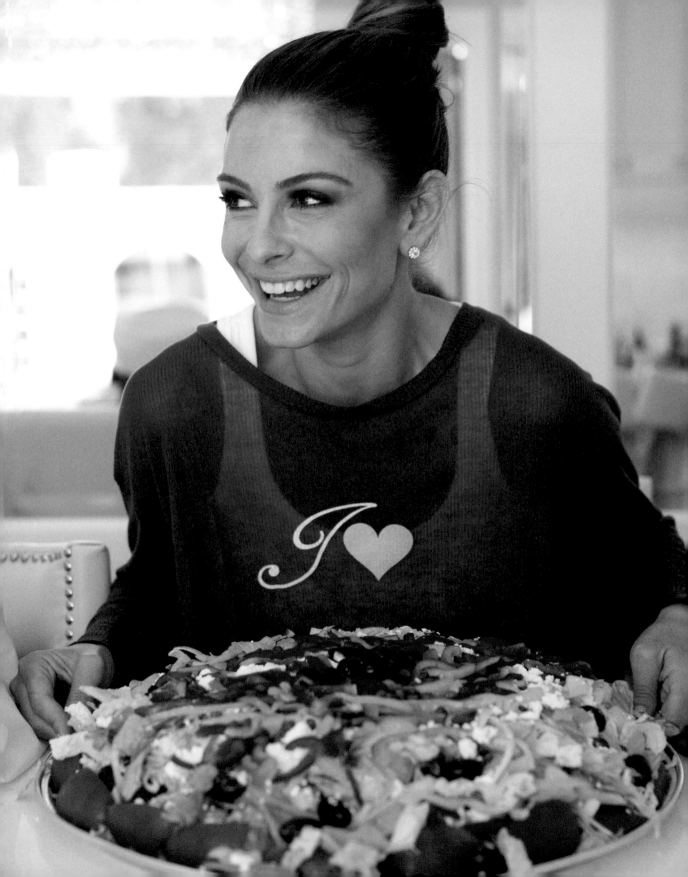

EveryGirl
MAKES LUNCH

Lunchtime is the eternal dilemma for EveryGirl. I know I need—even *want*—to eat a healthy lunch, but time is always tight and it's just so easy to grab a slice of pizza or pull up to the drive-through window. You really have to do a bit of planning to ensure a nutritious midday meal. I've come up with some go-to, portable, packable meals, some of which I can make in the morning (or even the night before). I've also included some special lunch recipes for weekends, when you might have more time to prepare and devote to sitting down to eat.

For any sandwich recipe in this section, you can substitute a wrap, pita, or even lettuce in place of the sliced bread.

My previous book, *The EveryGirl's Guide to Diet and Fitness*, includes many tips and tricks for preparing food you can eat on the go, but here's a quick recap:

- The more prep you do, the easier, healthier, and more cost-effective lunch will be. You also gain more control over your diet. This is especially handy if you are weight-conscious and certainly if you are health-conscious. Prepping also saves you time and stress over what you're going to do for lunch.

- Sundays are great days to whip up a bunch of meals for the week. Also, on nights while watching your favorite TV shows, you can pop in and out of the kitchen to prep meals for the next day.

- Investing in some glass or Tupperware stackable containers with lids is a must. They're great for grab-and-go meals to bring to the office or with you when you have to travel. I even transport food in resealable plastic bags, because I have a habit of forgetting to bring the Tupperware home!

- Unless you have an important lunchtime meeting, try to bring your lunch to work. Doing so saves you time and money, and that way you'll avoid the temptation of ordering pizza for lunch!

Three-Bean Power Salad

SERVES 6 TO 8   This recipe is diabetic-friendly and gluten-free!

Bring this colorful salad to your next picnic or potluck—it's the perfect make-ahead dish and it tastes even better the next day. For heartier appetites, fold in a cup or two of cooked shredded chicken.

¼ cup extra-virgin olive oil

¼ cup white wine or apple-cider vinegar

2 teaspoons Italian spice mixture or chopped fresh thyme

1 teaspoon Dijon mustard

Salt and black pepper

1 can (10 ounces) chickpeas, drained and rinsed

1 can (10 ounces) red kidney beans, drained and rinsed

1 can (8 ounces) low-sodium green beans, drained and rinsed

2 scallions, thinly sliced

1 stalk celery, thinly sliced

½ red pepper, cut into small dice

½ cup chopped fresh parsley or dill

1. In a large serving bowl, whisk the olive oil, vinegar, spice mixture, mustard, and salt and pepper to taste until blended.

2. Fold in the chickpeas, kidney beans, green beans, scallions, celery, red pepper, and parsley.

3. Refrigerate for at least 6 hours before serving.

EveryGirl
TIP: Traditionally, this dish is made with canned green beans. If that's not your thing, fresh green beans are a nice alternative. You don't even need to cook them first.

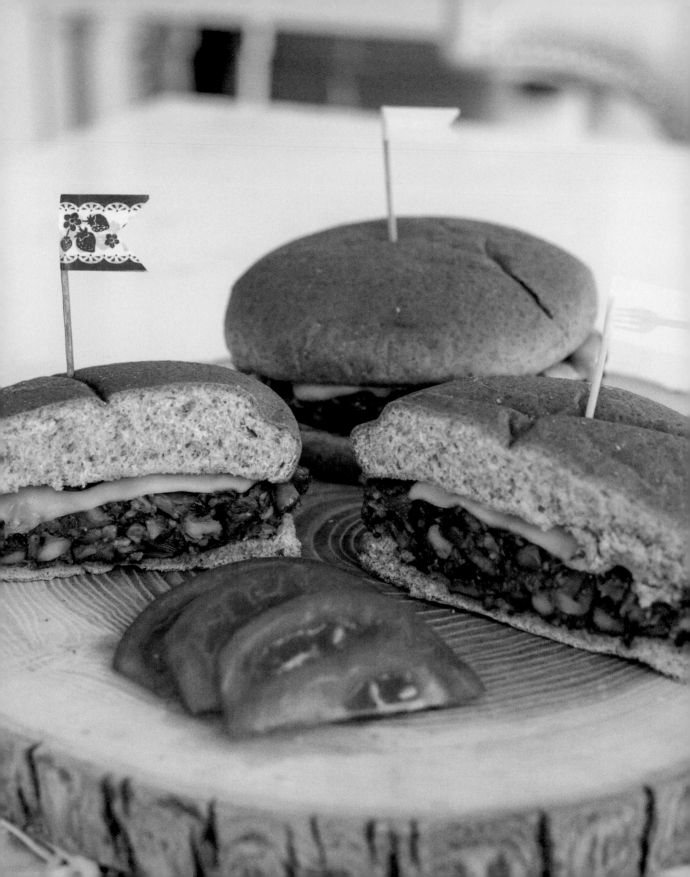

Portobello Mushroom Burger with Melted Gruyère on a Multigrain Bun

MAKES 4   Without the bun, this recipe is diabetic-friendly! **D**

These "burgers" are great if you are hosting a cookout and have some vegetarians coming. I promise, the non-vegetarians will want to try them too, so make a few extra and cut them in half! I think it's the combination of earthy mushrooms and sharp Gruyère that makes these so deliciously different and irresistible.

4 tablespoons olive oil

1 medium onion, chopped

3 portobello mushrooms, finely chopped

2 cloves garlic, minced

Salt and black pepper

1 large egg

½ cup walnuts, finely chopped

½ cup chopped fresh parsley

¼ cup bread crumbs

4 slices (4 ounces) Gruyère or Swiss cheese

4 multigrain or gluten-free buns

EveryGirl
TIP: Feel free to ditch the bun or omit the cheese, depending on your mood. If you want to, you can also use lettuce instead of the bun for a lower-calorie meal. Whatever you do, handle the burgers very carefully to keep the patties together.

1. Warm 2 tablespoons of the oil in a large skillet over medium-low heat. Cook the onion, mushrooms, garlic, and salt and pepper to taste until the mushrooms are soft, stirring.

2. In a large bowl, combine the egg, mushroom mixture, walnuts, parsley, and bread crumbs. Form 4 patties, using about ½ cup per patty.

3. Warm the remaining 2 tablespoons oil in the same skillet over medium-high heat. Cook the patties for 5 minutes on each side, or until browned. Lay a slice of cheese on top of each burger and continue to cook until melted.

4. Serve the burgers with the buns.

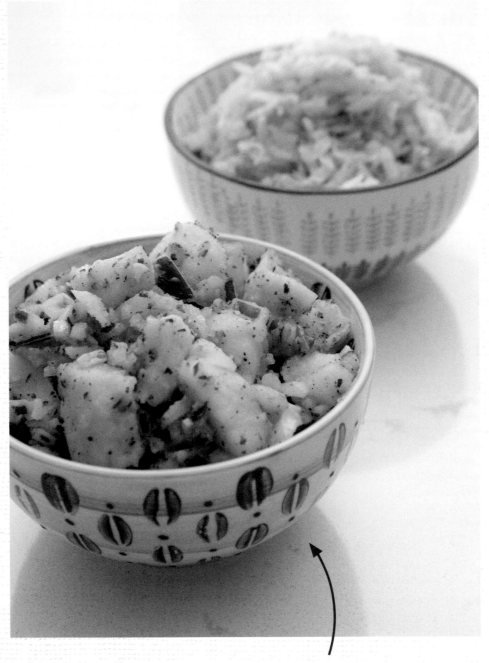

I bring my mom's potato salad to work with me all the time, and this cabbage salad recipe completely changed my mind about cabbage (I used to not like it at all). I think these two salads would make great side dishes for dinner as well.

Litsa's Potato Salad

SERVES 4

3 large russet potatoes
1 large red onion, finely chopped
1 tablespoon oregano
½ cup olive oil
⅓ cup red wine vinegar
Salt and black pepper

EveryGirl
TIP: To make this a healthy-carb meal, use Red Bliss potatoes and peel them.

1. Bake the potatoes for 12 minutes in the microwave. Peel and cut into chunks while they are hot, and place in a large bowl.

2. Mix in the red onion, oregano, olive oil, vinegar, and salt and pepper to taste.

Litsa's Cabbage Salad

SERVES 6   This recipe is diabetic-friendly and gluten-free!

1 tablespoon sea salt
1 small head of green cabbage, finely shredded
½ cup olive oil
¼ cup fresh lemon juice
2 tablespoons minced fresh garlic
Black pepper

EveryGirl
TIP: It's best to make this the night before, so it has time to marinate.

1. Add the sea salt to the shredded cabbage and work it into the cabbage with your hands, place the cabbage in a strainer with a bowl underneath, and squeeze the cabbage to drain the excess water. Leave in the fridge for 30 minutes (or overnight).

2. Add the olive oil, lemon juice, and garlic, and work through with your hands. Season with pepper to taste.

3. Transfer to a serving bowl when ready to eat.

Fancy Tuna Salad

SERVES 4   This recipe is diabetic-friendly and gluten-free!

Everyone loves my mom's tuna salad. She always makes a huge batch so we don't have to fight over who gets it in our house. I like to eat it plain and sometimes even drizzle a little vinegar on top. Or wrap it in lettuce.

¼ cup extra-virgin olive oil

2 tablespoons white wine or rice wine vinegar or fresh lemon juice

2 cloves garlic, minced

½ teaspoon minced fresh oregano

Salt and black pepper

1 small can (3 ounces) solid albacore tuna packed in water, drained

1 small carrot, shredded

½ small red onion, thinly sliced into rings

¼ cup crumbled feta cheese

½ green bell pepper, cut into thin strips

½ red bell pepper, cut into thin strips

5 green or red seedless grapes, cut into halves

½ small cucumber, diced (about ½ cup)

¼ cup chopped walnuts

TIP: This salad is packed with lots of colors and flavors and many more ingredients than I usually use. Of course, you can add and subtract as you like— using whatever vegetable, cheese, herb, or nut you happen to have. Remove the feta for a lower-calorie tuna dish.

1. In a large serving bowl, whisk together the oil, vinegar, garlic, oregano, and salt and pepper to taste until combined.

2. Add the tuna, carrot, red onion, feta, bell peppers, grapes, cucumber, and walnuts; toss to coat.

Crabmeat Sandwich

SERVES 2 This recipe is diabetic-friendly and, if you use gluten-free bread, it's gluten-free as well.

You can serve this crabmeat salad atop lettuce and garnish with chopped tomatoes, if you aren't in the mood for a sandwich.

¼ cup plain nonfat Greek yogurt
1 teaspoon fresh lemon juice
½ teaspoon Dijon mustard
Salt and black pepper
1 container (6 ounces) crabmeat, drained (you can find it in the
    refrigerator section of your supermarket, or buy it fresh)
¼ cup chopped celery
4 slices whole-grain or gluten-free bread, toasted
1 small tomato, thinly sliced
2 leaves Boston, Bibb, or romaine lettuce

1. In a large bowl, whisk together the yogurt, lemon juice, mustard, and salt and pepper to taste. Fold in the crabmeat and celery.

2. Make a sandwich with the crabmeat mixture, bread, tomato, and lettuce.

Balsamic Cherry Tomato Salad

SERVES 2   This recipe is diabetic-friendly and gluten-free!

So simple, so easy, so good. A pint of cherry tomatoes is that little plastic container you'll find in most markets. Just for fun, try using multicolored cherry tomatoes in this dish.

2 tablespoons extra-virgin olive oil

1 tablespoon balsamic vinegar

1 clove garlic, minced

½ small shallot, minced (about 1 tablespoon)

Salt and black pepper

1 tiny dash of sugar (evens out the bitter taste of the balsamic vinegar)

1 pint cherry tomatoes, halved

3 handfuls baby kale leaves or chopped romaine lettuce

2 tablespoons minced fresh basil leaves

1. In a large serving bowl, whisk the oil, vinegar, garlic, shallot, salt and pepper to taste, and a tiny dash of sugar.

2. Add the cherry tomatoes, kale, and basil; toss to coat.

Turkey-Cranberry Flatbread Wrap

SERVES 1

Turkey and cranberries aren't just for Thanksgiving!

- 1 tablespoon whipped cream cheese
- 2 tablespoons chopped sweetened dried cranberries
- 1 whole-grain or gluten-free wrap or tortilla
- 2 slices (about 2 ounces) turkey
- A few leaves of baby lettuce or baby arugula

1. In a small bowl, combine the cream cheese and cranberries.

2. Spread the cream cheese mixture on the wrap. Top with the turkey and lettuce, and roll up.

EveryGirl
TIP: For ease in spreading, use whipped cream cheese. If you love my EveryGirl Feta-Avocado Dip (page 151) as much as I do, use a tablespoon of that in place of the cream cheese.

Farmers' Market Pasta

SERVES 4 — If you use whole wheat pasta, one serving of this recipe makes a diabetic-friendly meal!

Use whole-wheat pasta if you want this to fit into the "good carb" category. I try to focus on "good carbs" more and more these days, as diabetes runs in my family.

½ pound penne or ziti pasta (regular, whole-wheat, or gluten-free)
¼ cup olive oil
1 medium onion, diced
1 medium zucchini, diced
1 yellow squash, diced
1 red bell pepper, diced
1 green bell pepper, diced
3 cloves garlic, minced
4 medium tomatoes, diced
Salt and black pepper

1. Cook the pasta according to the package directions. Drain, reserving ½ cup of the pasta cooking water.

2. Warm the oil in a large skillet over medium heat. Cook the onion for 5 minutes, stirring.

3. Add all the vegetables and cook for 10 minutes, stirring.

4. Transfer to a large serving bowl; toss with the pasta and pasta cooking water as needed. Season with salt and pepper to taste.

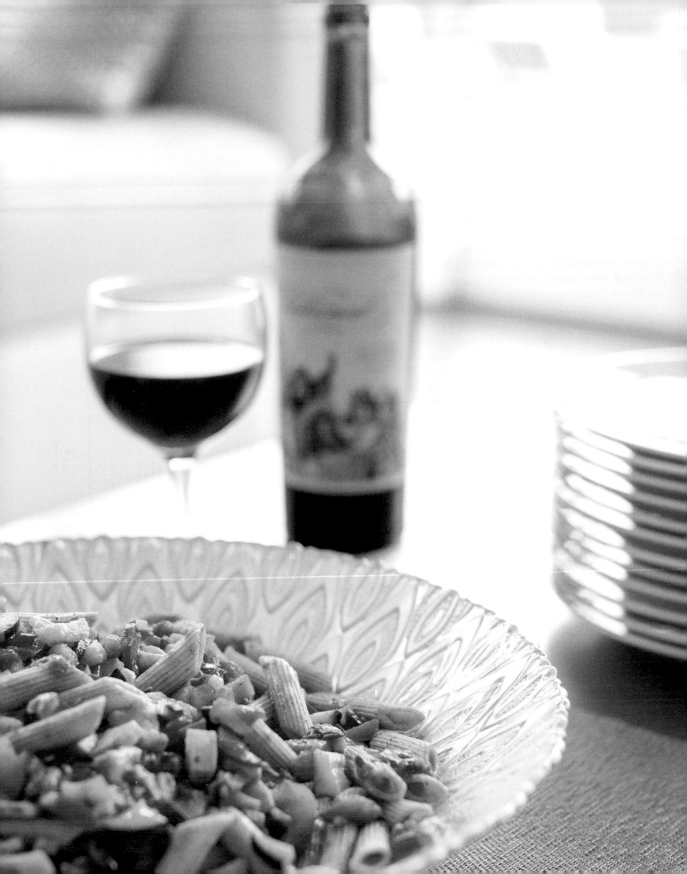

Grilled Chicken–Greek Salad Pita Pocket

SERVES 2

Use a low-carb pita and this recipe is diabetic-friendly!

This lunch looks and tastes like summer to me, but I enjoy it all year round.

Chicken
1 tablespoon olive oil
2 teaspoons chopped fresh oregano
Salt and black pepper
½ pound chicken tenders

Salad
1 tablespoon extra-virgin olive oil
1 tablespoon fresh lemon juice (from 1 lemon)
Salt and black pepper
2 cups chopped romaine lettuce
½ cup crumbled feta cheese
1 medium tomato, sliced
½ cucumber, diced
2 large pita breads

1. In a resealable plastic bag, combine the oil and oregano, and salt and pepper to taste. Add the chicken, seal the bag, and turn to coat. Marinate for at least 30 minutes in the refrigerator or up to 12 hours.

2. Grill the chicken on a medium-hot grill or a grill pan until just cooked through, turning occasionally. (You can also use a George Foreman Grill if you have one.)

3. For the salad: In a large bowl, whisk the oil, lemon juice, and salt and pepper to taste. Add the grilled chicken, lettuce, feta, tomato, and cucumber; toss to coat. Stuff the mixture into the pita.

EveryGirl

TIP: For the best flavor, use extra-virgin olive oil for salads and uncooked dishes and use the less-expensive regular olive oil for cooking.

EveryGirl

TIP: There's no need to peel the cucumber if you are dicing it into small pieces, as in this salad.

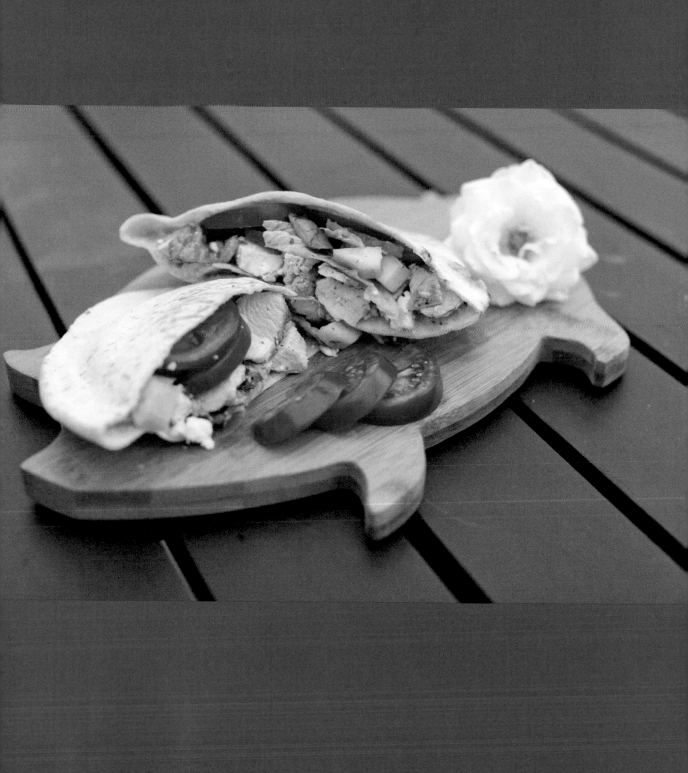

Romaine Chopped Salad

SERVES 1 TO 2   This recipe is diabetic-friendly and gluten-free!

This bright crisp salad works as a big main dish for one or a small side dish for two. Can't handle raw onion? The salad is still delicious without it.

1 tablespoon extra-virgin olive oil

2 teaspoons fresh lemon juice

¼ teaspoon Dijon mustard

Salt and black pepper

2 cups chopped romaine lettuce

¼ cup minced red onion

1 small tomato, diced

1 small cucumber, diced

¼ cup drained canned chickpeas

1. In a large serving bowl, whisk together the oil, lemon juice, and mustard, and salt and pepper to taste.

2. Add the lettuce, onion, tomato, cucumber, and chickpeas; toss to coat.

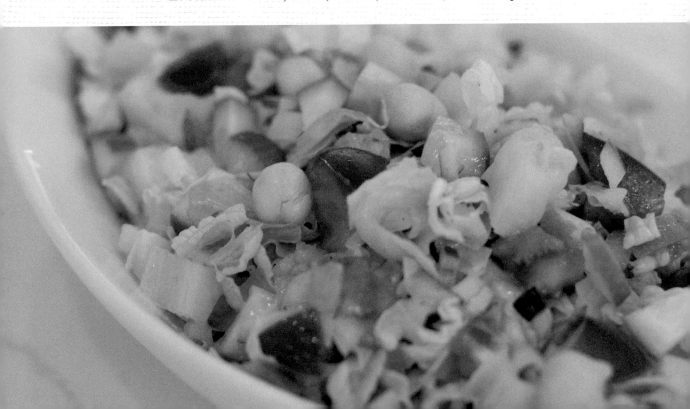

Caramelized Veggie Flatbreads

SERVES 4

There are all kinds of flatbreads now available at the supermarket, even gluten-free options. Experiment until you find the one you like best.

2 tablespoons olive oil
1 small red bell pepper, thinly sliced
1 small green bell pepper, thinly sliced
1 small yellow bell pepper, thinly sliced
1 small onion, thinly sliced
Salt and black pepper
4 pieces flatbread, naan bread, or large pita bread
4 tablespoons part-skim ricotta cheese
8 large basil leaves, thinly sliced

EveryGirl
TIP: The easiest way to slice basil is to stack the leaves, then roll the stack into a tight cylinder. Thinly slice the cylinder crosswise.

1. Warm the oil in a large nonstick skillet over medium-low heat. Add the sliced peppers and onion; cook for 20 minutes, or until softened and caramelized, stirring often. Season with salt and pepper to taste.

2. Toast or warm the bread; spread the ricotta cheese on the warm bread.

3. Top with the veggies and sliced basil.

Grilled Chicken Tenders and Baby Arugula Salad

SERVES 4   Leave out the dried cranberries and this recipe is diabetic-friendly. **D** **GF**
                     Even with the cranberries, it's gluten-free!

Greens and lean protein are a terrific lunchtime combination and this simple vinaigrette works perfectly with both.

Chicken

3 tablespoons olive oil
3 cloves garlic, peeled and crushed
Salt and black pepper
1 tablespoon paprika
1 pound chicken tenders

Salad

2 tablespoons extra-virgin olive oil
1 tablespoon fresh lemon juice or white-wine vinegar
Salt and black pepper
4 handfuls baby arugula (about 8 cups)
2 medium tomatoes, sliced
½ cup sunflower seeds (salted or unsalted)
½ cup sweetened dried cranberries

1. In a resealable plastic bag or a glass bowl, combine the oil, the garlic, salt and pepper to taste, and paprika. Add the chicken, seal the bag, and turn to coat. Let marinate for at least 30 minutes, or up to 12 hours.

2. Grill the chicken on a medium-hot grill or in a grill pan until just cooked through, turning occasionally. (Discard the marinade.)

EveryGirl

TIP: Delicate meats like skinless chicken breasts shouldn't marinate for longer than 12 hours or so, or the meat might get mushy. Always marinate in the refrigerator.

3. For the salad, in a large bowl, whisk the oil, lemon juice, and salt and pepper to taste. Add the arugula, tomatoes, sunflower seeds, and cranberries; toss to coat with the dressing.

4. Top the salad with the grilled chicken.

EveryGirl

TIP: As with most salads, wait to toss the greens until just before serving. If making this in advance, keep the components separate until lunchtime. Use any green lettuce leaf you prefer.

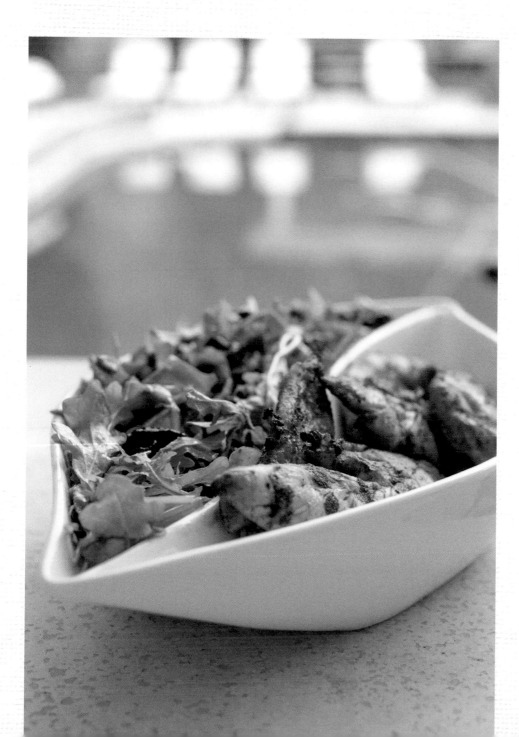

Potato, Chickpea, and Kale Soup

SERVES 4

A healthy soup with some hearty texture!

2 tablespoons olive oil

2 medium red or Yukon Gold potatoes, cut into small dice

Salt and black pepper

1 medium onion, chopped

2 cloves garlic, minced

1 (14½-ounce) can chickpeas, drained

½ small bunch kale, stems removed and leaves coarsely chopped

½ cup grated Parmesan cheese

EveryGirl

TIP: Although a bit more expensive, fresh Parmesan gives a much better flavor to this soup than grated Parmesan in a container.

1. Warm the oil in a medium saucepan over medium-low heat.

2. Add the potatoes, salt and pepper to taste, and cook for 5 minutes, or until browned, stirring. Add the onion and garlic; cook for 5 minutes, stirring.

3. Add the chickpeas and 2½ cups water; bring to a simmer.

4. Add the kale; cook for 10 minutes, or until wilted.

5. Garnish the servings with the cheese.

Cranberry-Chicken Salad

SERVES 3 TO 4

Skip the dried cranberries and this recipe is diabetic friendly. **D**
Even with them, it's gluten-free!

Feel free to make this salad your own. Substitute apple for the cranberries, almonds for the sunflower seeds, scallions for the red onion. You get the idea!

- ¼ cup fresh raspberries
- ¼ cup extra-virgin olive oil
- 3 tablespoons apple-cider vinegar
- Salt and black pepper
- 2 cups diced cooked white-meat chicken
- 1 stalk celery, thinly sliced
- ½ cup diced red bell pepper
- ½ cup sweetened dried cranberries
- ½ cup salted sunflower seeds
- 2 tablespoons diced red onion, as desired

1. In a medium bowl, mash the raspberries with a fork. Whisk in the oil and vinegar, and salt and pepper to taste.

2. Add the diced chicken, celery, red pepper, cranberries, sunflower seeds, and onion. Toss to coat.

EveryGirl
TIP: Don't have any cooked chicken? Pick up a rotisserie chicken and use the breast meat. Remember to remove the skin.

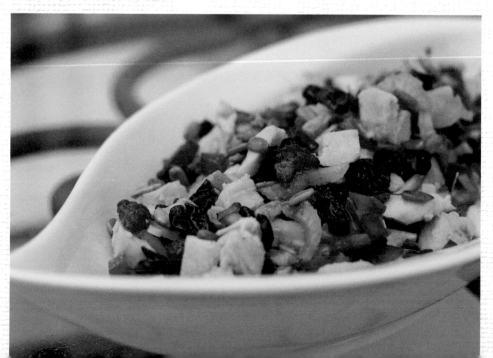

Kale and Lemon Oil Pizza

SERVES 2 TO 3

If your friends like pizza, why not throw a pizza party? Get a bunch of ready-made crusts and set an area of your counter with different toppings and cheeses. I like to have ricotta, mozzarella (fresh, if possible), feta for a Greek-style pizza, veggie toppings, basil, oregano, tomato sauce, and any meats you would like to experiment with! It's fun for everyone!

Vegetable oil and cornmeal, for the pan

1 pound prepared pizza dough

1 tablespoon olive oil

½ bunch (about 6 ounces) kale, stems removed and leaves coarsely chopped

2 cloves garlic, minced

2 tablespoons fresh lemon juice (from 1 lemon)

¾ cup (3 ounces) shredded mozzarella cheese

Salt and black pepper

2 teaspoons pine nuts

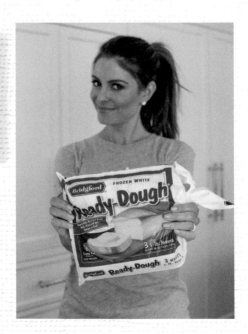
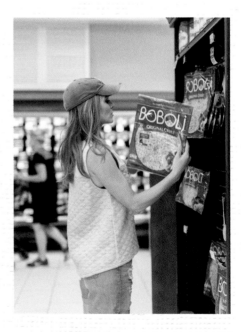

1. Preheat the oven to 425°F.

2. Lightly oil a large baking sheet (or 2 small baking sheets) with vegetable oil and sprinkle with cornmeal.

3. Using a sharp knife, cut the pizza dough in half. Using your hands, stretch each piece into an oval shape, about 10 by 6 inches. Place on the prepared sheet(s).

4. Warm the olive oil in a large skillet over medium-low heat. Add the kale and garlic; cook for 6 minutes, or until wilted, stirring. Stir in the lemon juice.

5. Spread the kale mixture over the pizza dough and sprinkle with the cheese. Bake for 16 minutes, or until the edges of the crust are golden and the cheese melts.

6. Season with salt and pepper to taste and garnish with the pine nuts.

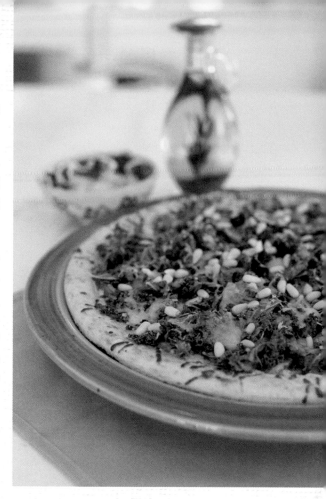

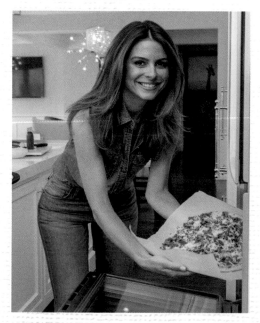

Garden Pasta Salad with Tuna

SERVES 4

I have so many lemon trees in my yard and always try to incorporate the fruit into everything! When I was younger, I would eat the lemons as is! They have so many health benefits, like aiding in digestion and respiratory disorders, but are also great for skin, hair, and even weight loss.

½ pound small shell pasta (regular, whole-wheat, or rice)

½ cup mayonnaise or plain Greek yogurt (choose whatever mayo you like, fat-free or regular for more taste)

3 tablespoons fresh lemon juice (from 2 lemons)

1 can (6 ounces) solid albacore tuna packed in water

½ cup shredded carrots or diced red bell pepper or cucumber

2 stalks celery, thinly sliced

Big handful of chopped lettuce leaves

3 tablespoons chopped fresh chives

Salt

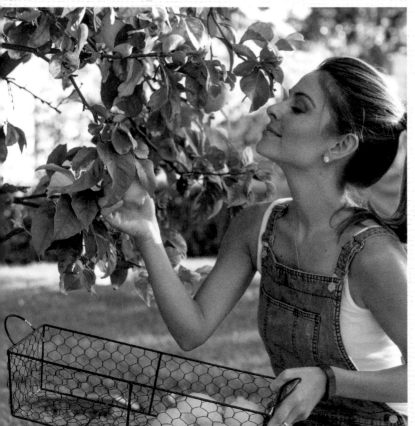

1. Cook the pasta according to the package directions. Drain.

2. In a large serving bowl, whisk the mayonnaise and lemon juice. Fold in the tuna. Add the carrots, celery, lettuce, and chives. Season to taste with salt.

EveryGirl CELEBRITY COOKING MOMENT

The greatest honor I've ever had in cooking was being able to create dishes for celebrity cooking icon Rachael Ray! She is one of the sweetest, most supportive women in our business. Every time I go on her show, my mom and I bring recipes from our kitchen. Rachael always takes the time to sample and comment on them and is always so grateful and appreciative. I can't thank her enough for all the support she has given me over the years.

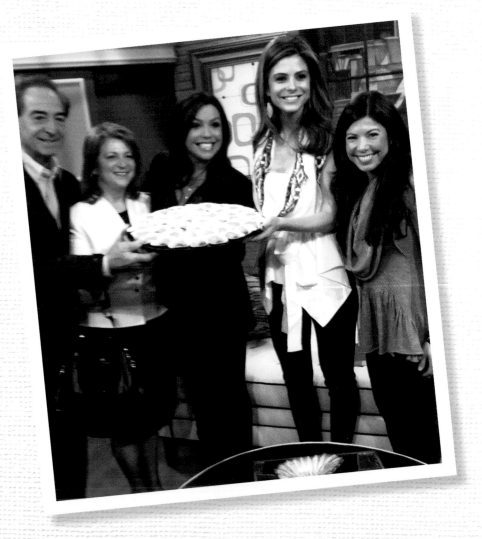

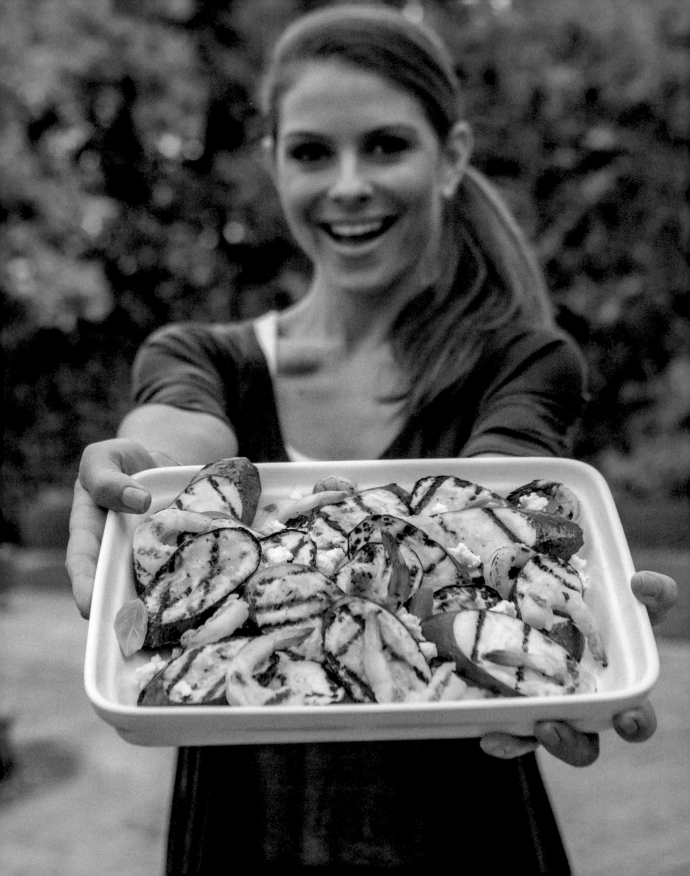

EveryGirl

COOKS DINNER

Dinner is the most important meal of the day—not so much nutritionally speaking, but certainly emotionally. I used to be so amazed that after she had put in a long day at work, my mother still had the energy to cook a delicious dinner for the family. I realize now just how important those evening meals were—both to reconnect with the family and to provide nutritious from-the-heart meals. In addition, our greatest memories back then as mother and daughter came from those days we cooked together. It's a great bonding experience that I hope to share with my kids, one day.

These days, whenever possible, Kev and I try to cook dinners at home, too. We love leftovers and on some nights we cook up a double recipe, so we are all set the next night! Also, when sharing dinner at home with loved ones, we talk about what's going on in our lives and the news of the day. It is a healthy way for a couple or family to spend quality time together and to bond. Having everyone pitch in doesn't hurt, either! In our house, I cook and Kev cleans!

Eggplant and Zucchini

SERVES 6

This recipe is diabetic-friendly and gluten-free! **D** **GF**

This dish is so versatile. Serve as a side dish, a bed for grilled chicken or fish, a baguette topping, or a dip.

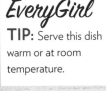

EveryGirl
TIP: Serve this dish warm or at room temperature.

3 tablespoons olive oil
1 eggplant, cut into ½-inch cubes
1 small onion, diced
1 zucchini, cut into ½-inch cubes
1 red bell pepper, cut into ½-inch cubes
1 can (8 ounces) diced tomatoes
¾ cup tomato juice or V8 Vegetable Juice
¼ cup red wine vinegar
¼ cup prepared or homemade pesto

1. Warm 2 tablespoons of the oil in a large skillet over medium-high heat. Add the eggplant; cook for 10 minutes, stirring often. Transfer to a bowl.

2. Add the remaining 1 tablespoon oil to the skillet over medium heat. Add the onion, zucchini, red pepper, and tomatoes; cook for 8 minutes, or until the vegetables are softened.

3. Stir in the tomato juice, vinegar, and browned eggplant. Simmer for 8 minutes, or until the juice thickens and the vegetables are cooked through.

4. Stir in the pesto.

One-Pan Pork Chops with Green Beans

SERVES 4   This recipe is diabetic-friendly and gluten-free!

I don't eat a lot of pork personally, but realized we didn't have many recipes for those who do. Mom's pork chops are definitely winners!

  4 tablespoons olive oil
  Juice of 1 lemon (about 3 tablespoons)
  2 tablespoons chopped fresh thyme
  4 cloves garlic, minced
  Salt and black pepper
  4 bone-in pork chops (each 1-inch thick)
  12 ounces green beans, trimmed

1. Preheat the oven to 450°F.

2. In a large bowl, combine 2 tablespoons of the oil, the lemon juice, thyme, garlic, and salt and pepper to taste. Add the pork chops and turn to coat.

3. On a large, rimmed baking sheet, toss the green beans with the remaining 2 tablespoons oil and salt and pepper to taste. Spread in an even layer on the baking sheet.

4. Nestle the pork chops among the beans. Place in the oven and roast for 25 minutes, turning the pork chops once, until the vegetables are tender and the chops are just cooked through.

EveryGirl
TIP: Prepping green beans is a snap—literally. Just snap off the stem end of each bean. If they are super long, snap the beans in half as well.

Crustless Chicken Pot Pie

SERVES 6 TO 8

If you use whole-wheat bread crumbs and whole-wheat flour, this recipe is diabetic-friendly.

I know most of our dishes are healthy, but they can't all be! And who doesn't love a delicious chicken pot pie.

EveryGirl

TIP: Whenever you are adding frozen peas to a cooked dish, there's no need to thaw them.

1¼ pounds boneless, skinless chicken breast halves

1 cup frozen peas

4 tablespoons (½ stick) unsalted butter

1 onion, thinly sliced

3 carrots, peeled and thinly sliced

¼ cup all-purpose flour

1 cup nonfat milk

Salt and black papper

⅓ cup bread crumbs

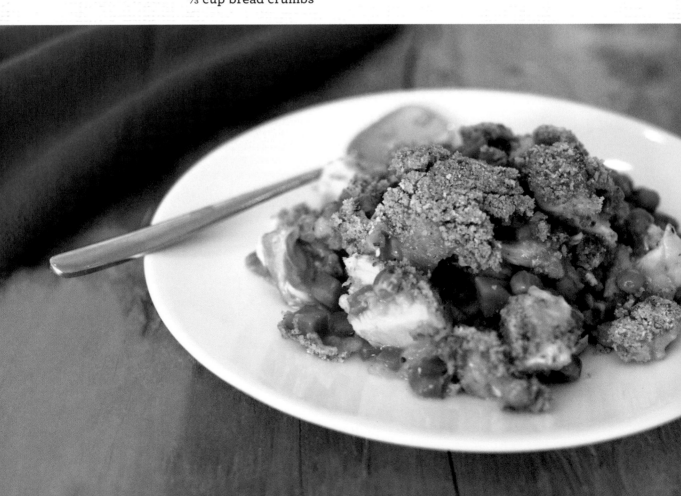

1. Preheat the oven to 350°F.

2. Lay the chicken breasts in a medium saucepan; cover with water by at least 1 inch. Bring to a boil over medium-high heat. Reduce the heat to low; cover and simmer for 10 minutes, or until the chicken is just cooked through. (Reserve 1½ cups of the poaching liquid; discard the rest.)

3. Dice the chicken. In a 2-quart casserole, combine the diced chicken and peas.

4. Melt the butter in a medium saucepan over low heat. Cook the onion and carrots for 10 minutes, stirring. Sprinkle in the flour and stir until a paste is formed.

5. Very slowly pour in the milk and the warm poaching liquid, stirring the whole time, until a thick sauce forms. (This can take as long as 10 minutes.)

6. Fold the sauce into the chicken mixture in the casserole. Season with salt and pepper to taste. Cover the pan with foil; bake for 15 minutes.

7. Uncover, sprinkle with the bread crumbs, and bake for 15 minutes, or until hot.

EveryGirl
TIP: Save time by using white meat cut from a rotisserie chicken rather than cooking chicken yourself. If you do that, you won't have the poaching broth, so use 2½ cups milk or canned chicken broth to make the sauce.

White Bean–Stuffed Pork

This recipe is diabetic-friendly and gluten-free!

If you don't like pork, this recipe works just as well with beef tenderloin or with a pounded chicken breast.

1½ pounds pork tenderloin
¼ cup olive oil
1 large onion, thinly sliced
1 medium carrot, peeled and thinly sliced
¾ cup drained canned white beans
2 cloves garlic, minced
1 teaspoon chopped fresh thyme, or ½ teaspoon dried thyme
Salt and black pepper
Baking twine or toothpicks

EveryGirl

TIP: If all the filling doesn't fit inside the pork, save it and add it to the skillet in the last few minutes of cooking, to warm. Serve alongside the pork slices.

1. Preheat the oven to 400°F.

2. To butterfly the tenderloin, lay it out on a cutting board. Make a lengthwise cut down through the center of the meat, stopping before you get to the board, so that you have a hinge to open and stuff.

3. Warm 2 tablespoons of the oil in a large cast-iron or ovenproof skillet over medium-low heat. Add the onion, carrot, beans, garlic, thyme, and salt and pepper to taste, and cook for 10 minutes, stirring.

4. Spread the filling over the flattened pork; close the hinge to cover the filling. Use twine or toothpicks to hold the pork together. Season the pork with more salt and pepper.

5. Warm the remaining 2 tablespoons oil in the same skillet over medium-high heat. Brown the pork on all sides, about 8 minutes. Transfer the skillet to the oven and roast the pork for 22 minutes, or until an instant-read thermometer inserted into the thickest part registers 145°F.

6. Remove to a cutting board; let rest for 5 minutes before slicing.

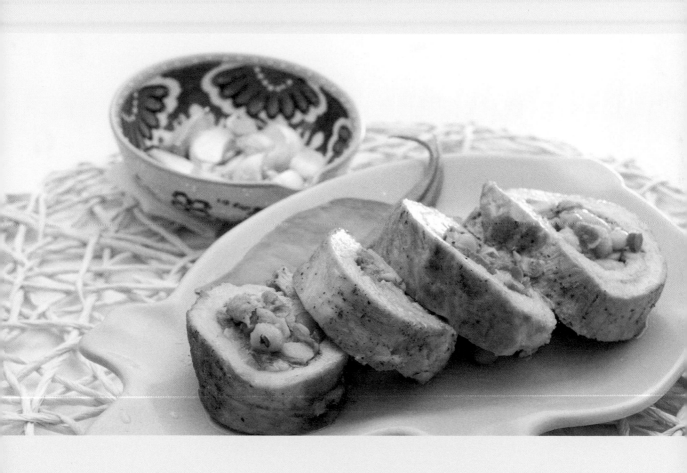

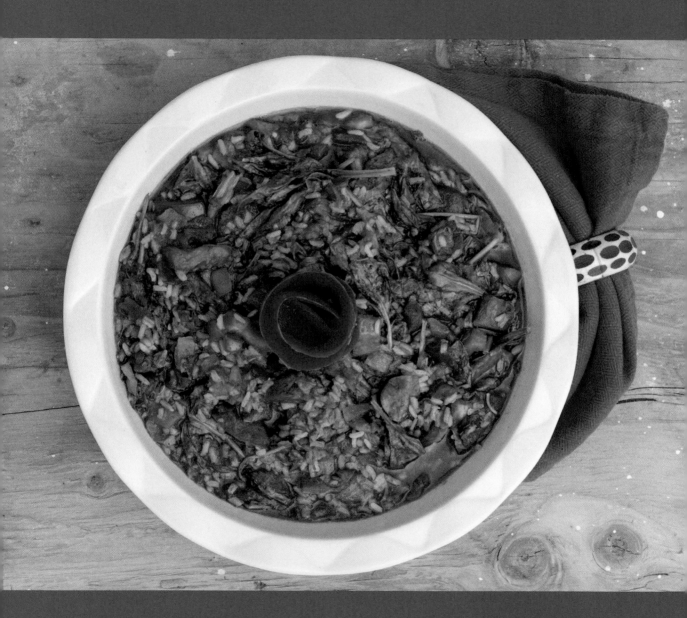

Spinach and Rice

SERVES 2   If you use brown rice, this recipe is diabetic-friendly.
Either way it's gluten-free!

*It might seem like I'm using a lot of spinach in this recipe, but it cooks down
so dramatically that you have to start with a lot to make this much.*

2 tablespoons olive oil

1 large onion, diced

2 packages baby spinach

1 tablespoon dried mint

Salt and black pepper

4 large tomatoes, diced

1 cup cooked brown or white rice

EveryGirl
TIP: When you first
add the spinach to the
skillet, let it sit for a
minute to soften, then
stir and cook.

1. Warm the oil in a medium saucepan over medium heat.

2. Cook the onion for 5 minutes, stirring.

3. Stir in the spinach, mint, and salt and pepper to taste.

4. Add the tomatoes and rice; cook for 5 minutes, to warm through.

Whole-Wheat Spaghetti with White-Wine Mushroom Sauce

SERVES 2   As long as you use whole-wheat pasta, this recipe is diabetic-friendly. Use gluten-free pasta and it's gluten-free!

I love going with whole-wheat pasta whenever I get the chance—and it's just as delicious, in my opinion!

½ pound whole-wheat spaghetti (or gluten-free)

2 tablespoons olive oil

18 ounces white or cremini mushrooms, stemmed and sliced

3 scallions, white and light green parts only, sliced

2 cloves garlic, minced

Salt and black pepper

½ cup white wine

½ cup grated Parmesan cheese

¼ cup chopped fresh parsley

EveryGirl

TIP: Try to purchase mushrooms loose, rather than wrapped in a box. They are usually much fresher. Remember to snap off the stems before cooking.

EveryGirl

TIP: All of the alcohol in the wine cooks off, but if you prefer not to use wine, you can substitute with chicken broth.

1. Cook the pasta according to the package directions. Drain.

2. Meanwhile, warm the oil in a large skillet over medium heat. Add the mushrooms, scallions, garlic, and salt and pepper to taste. Cook, stirring, for 5 minutes, or until the mushrooms are softened and give off their liquid.

3. Add the wine; cook, stirring, for about 4 minutes, until the alcohol evaporates.

4. In a large bowl, combine the cooked pasta, mushroom sauce, cheese, and parsley.

Balsamic-Marinated Grilled Flank Steak with Dilled Yogurt Sauce

SERVES 4   This recipe is diabetic-friendly and gluten-free!

You can adjust the marinating time longer depending on your schedule—even let the meat marinate overnight if you have time—but 30 minutes is the minimum.

Steak

1 tablespoon balsamic vinegar

1 tablespoon olive oil

1 clove garlic, minced

Salt and black pepper

1½ pounds flank steak

Sauce

3 tablespoons extra-virgin olive oil

3 tablespoons fresh lemon juice

½ teaspoon salt

1 small clove garlic, minced

2 tablespoons minced fresh dill

1 cup plain nonfat Greek yogurt

EveryGirl

TIP: Always let grilled meat rest for a few minutes before slicing it. And never slice meat on the grill. It will dry it out!

1. Preheat the grill to high.

2. In a large resealable bag, combine the vinegar, olive oil, garlic, and salt and pepper to taste. Add the steak; flip to coat. Refrigerate for at least 30 minutes or overnight, flipping the bag occasionally to coat the meat. Let sit at room temperature for 30 minutes before cooking.

3. Grill the steak to the desired doneness. Let rest for 10 minutes before slicing.

4. For the sauce: In a medium bowl, whisk the oil, the lemon juice, salt, garlic, and dill. Fold in the yogurt. Serve with the steak.

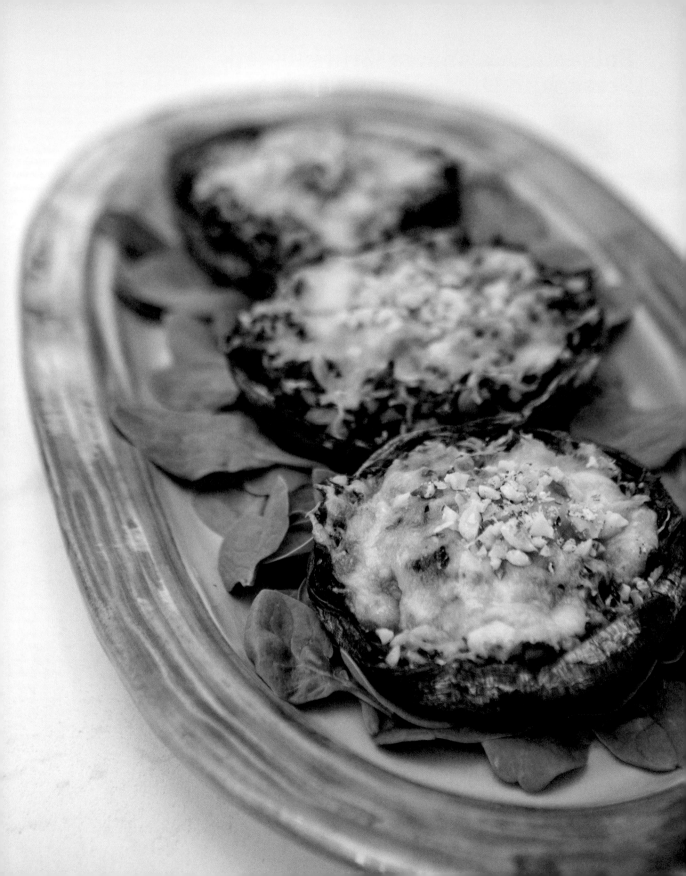

Spinach and Walnut–Stuffed Portobello Mushrooms

SERVES 4   This recipe is diabetic-friendly and gluten-free!

My favorite thing about Mom's recipes is that they are short on ingredients, for the most part, and short on instructions. That's why they're easy! These look so fancy and they are simple to make! Feel free to play with other ingredients the next time you make them. Make them your own!

4 portobello mushrooms

1 tablespoon olive oil

1 small onion, diced

4 cups chopped spinach

3 cloves garlic, minced

¼ cup shredded mozzarella cheese

¼ cup chopped walnuts

EveryGirl
TIP: Baby spinach leaves and regular spinach can be used interchangeably in most recipes. Baby spinach is more expensive, but saves time because it doesn't need to be trimmed or washed.

1. Preheat the oven to 400°F.

2. Remove the stems from the mushrooms; coarsely chop the stems.

3. Warm the oil in a large skillet over medium heat. Add the chopped mushroom stems, onion, spinach, and garlic; cook for 8 minutes, or until softened, stirring.

4. Fill the mushroom caps and sprinkle with the cheese. Bake for 15 minutes, or until the mushrooms soften.

5. Transfer to a platter and top with the walnuts.

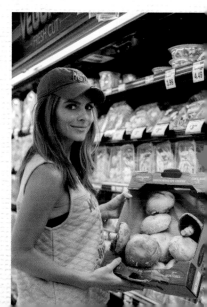

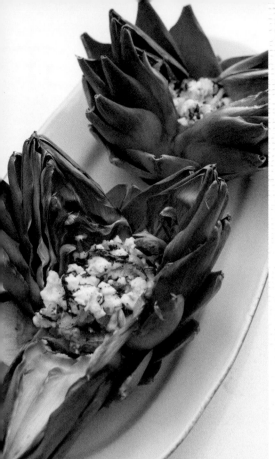

Double Cheese–Stuffed Artichokes

SERVES 4   This recipe is diabetic-friendly and gluten-free!

Okay, I know what you are thinking; this looks hard. I was intimidated, too, but today I love making these stuffed artichokes. All it takes is one try to remove your fear. This recipe is fairly simple and super impressive if you are entertaining. And, by the way, you will die when you taste it!

4 fresh or frozen whole artichokes, stems trimmed
2 tablespoons olive oil
1 small onion, chopped
3 cloves garlic, minced
½ cup chopped fresh parsley
½ cup crumbled feta cheese
Salt and black pepper
½ cup shredded mozzarella cheese

1. Bring a large pot of water to a boil over high heat. Add the artichokes to the simmering water (the water should go about halfway up the sides of the artichokes). Simmer for 35 minutes, or until the artichokes are tender.

EveryGirl
TIP: Since artichokes can be expensive, keep your eye out for store specials, which usually happen in the spring, when they are in season.

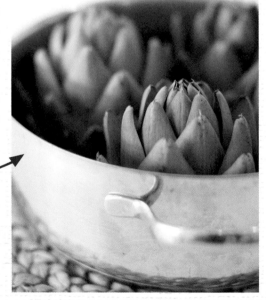

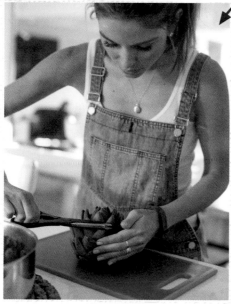

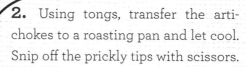

2. Using tongs, transfer the artichokes to a roasting pan and let cool. Snip off the prickly tips with scissors.

3. Using your fingers, pull back the center leaves, so the artichoke opens to reveal the inner leaves and fuzzy choke at the bottom. Using a small spoon, gently scrape out and discard the inedible choke.

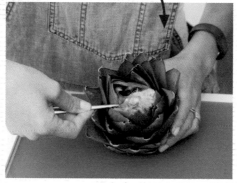

EveryGirl
TIP: Once you've removed the fuzzy choke and snipped off the prickly tips, you can eat the whole artichoke. Make sure you scoop out all the fuzzy parts, but be careful you don't take out the whole heart that's underneath. Just the fuzzies!

4. Preheat the oven to 400°F.

5. Warm the oil in a large skillet over medium heat. Cook the onion and garlic for 5 minutes, or until softened, stirring.

6. In a large bowl, combine the onion mixture, parsley, feta, and salt and pepper to taste.

7. Fill the artichoke centers with the onion mixture. Top with the shredded mozzarella. Bake for 15 minutes, or until warmed through and the cheese has melted.

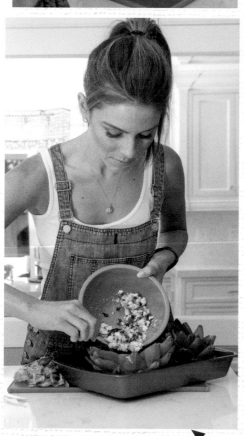

EVERYGIRL COOKS DINNER **99**

Eggplant-Tomato Casserole with Melted Feta

SERVES 4   This recipe is diabetic-friendly and gluten-free! **D** **GF**

This recipe is a great side dish for grilled steak or chicken. It also works as a warm dip for a dinner party.

¼ cup olive oil
1 medium eggplant, diced
1 can (7 ounces) diced tomatoes
2 cloves garlic, minced
3 tablespoons fresh lemon juice
2 tablespoons chopped fresh dill
Salt and black pepper
¾ cup crumbled feta cheese

1. Preheat the broiler.

2. Warm the oil in a large ovenproof skillet over medium-low heat. Add the eggplant and tomatoes; cook for 15 minutes, stirring to brown the eggplant on all sides.

3. Add the garlic, lemon juice, dill, and salt and pepper to taste, and cook for 1 minute, stirring occasionally. Remove from the heat; top with the feta.

4. Transfer the pan to the broiler. Broil for 2 minutes, or until the feta is warmed through and bubbling.

Beef and Pepper Stir-Fry

SERVES 4   This recipe is diabetic-friendly if you use brown rice, and it's gluten-free either way!

Although the stir-fry has a lot of ingredients, it's quick to put together and even quicker to cook.

¼ cup olive oil
1 medium onion, sliced
1 red bell pepper, sliced
1 green bell pepper, sliced
1 pound thinly sliced lean beef (see Tip)
2 cloves garlic, minced
1 can tomato sauce
Salt and black pepper
2 cups cooked brown rice, warmed (if desired)

1. Warm the oil in a large nonstick skillet over medium-high heat. Stir-fry the onion and the bell peppers.

2. Add the beef strips and garlic; stir-fry for 4 minutes. Add the tomato sauce and salt and pepper to taste; cook for 4 minutes, or until the beef is cooked through.

3. Serve with rice, if desired.

EveryGirl
TIP: Look for beef labeled "Beef for Stir-Fry" at the market.

Fancy Spinach-Stuffed Chicken

SERVES 4   This recipe is diabetic-friendly and gluten-free!

You'll need to use large chicken breast halves to hold all of the delicious filling for this recipe. And I'll bet this one becomes one of your go-to chicken dinner recipes!

2 tablespoons olive oil

1 small onion, diced

4 cups chopped spinach

2 cloves garlic, minced

Salt and black pepper

¼ cup cooked quinoa or brown rice

⅓ cup ricotta cheese

2 tablespoons pine nuts

2 large boneless, skinless chicken breast halves (about 7 ounces each), cut in half crosswise

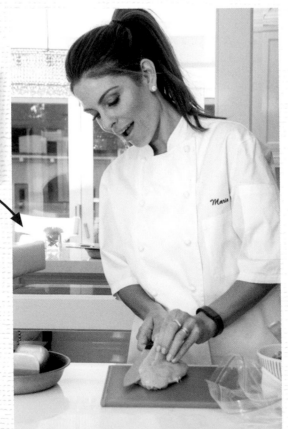

EveryGirl
TIP: To prep the chicken, use a sharp knife to horizontally slice each breast crosswise.

1. Preheat the oven to 400°F.

2. Warm 1 tablespoon of the oil in a large ovenproof skillet over medium heat. Add the onion, spinach, garlic, and salt and pepper to taste; cook for 6 minutes, stirring, until the onion is translucent and the spinach is wilted. Transfer to a bowl. Stir in the quinoa, ricotta, and pine nuts. Don't wash the skillet. Put the filling aside.

3. Place the chicken pieces in a resealable plastic bag. Using a mallet or the bottom of a pan, pound the pieces to about ¼ inch thick. Season the chicken with salt and pepper to taste.

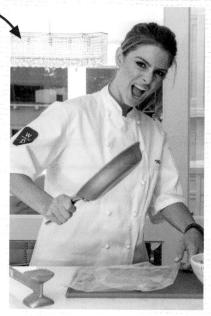

EveryGirl
TIP: Kitchen tongs are the best tool to gently lift and turn the chicken bundles.

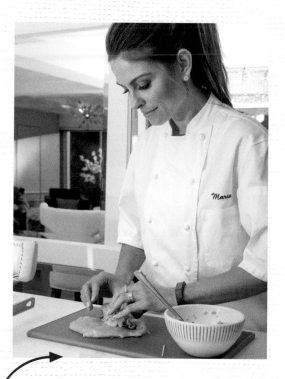

Voila!

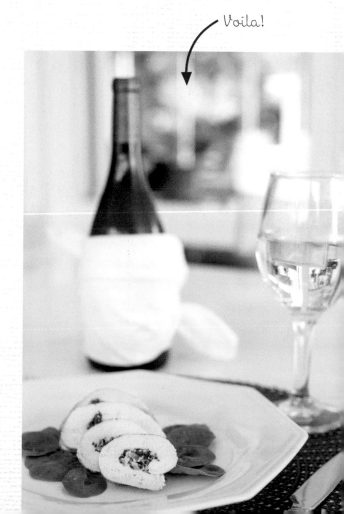

4. Divide the spinach mixture among the chicken pieces; roll the chicken into a tight cylinder. Use a toothpick to keep the rolls together.

5. Warm the remaining 1 tablespoon oil in the same skillet over medium-high heat. Cook the chicken bundles in the skillet for 10 minutes, turning to brown evenly.

6. Transfer the chicken bundles to a baking sheet and place in the oven. Cook for 12 minutes, until the chicken is cooked through and the filling is hot.

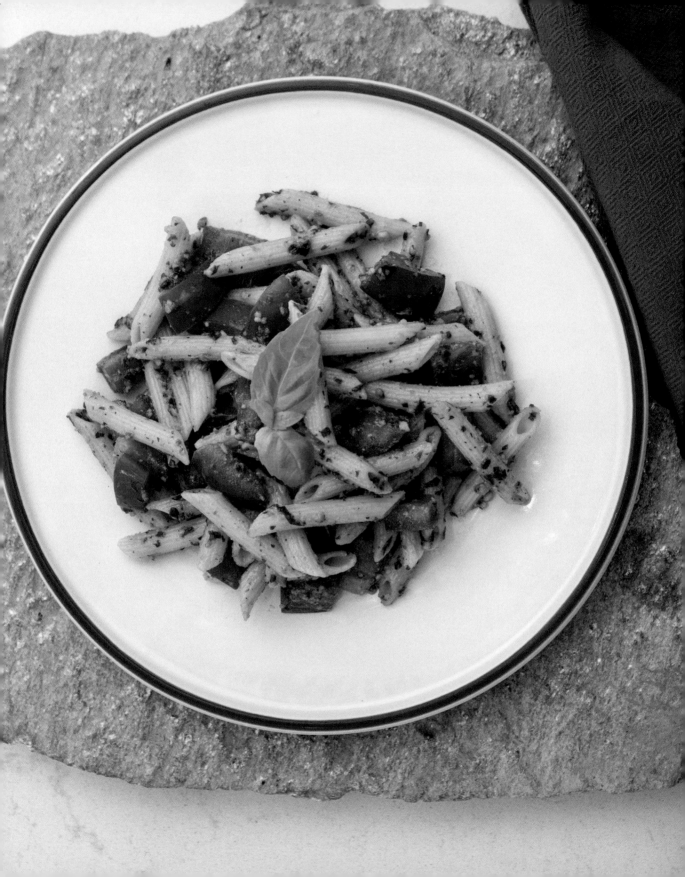

Everyone Loves Pasta Pesto with August Tomatoes

SERVES 4 TO 6

You can add more or less of any of these ingredients and taste-test as you go. In fact, I never use a recipe for my pesto and had to really pay attention in order to write this one down for you. Feel free to do as I usually do: Just put the ingredients in the blender and taste it. Have fun with it!

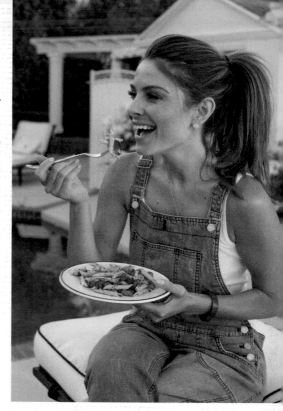

1 pound pasta of your choice

5 cups packed fresh basil

½ cup extra-virgin olive oil

6 tablespoons grated Parmesan cheese

⅓ cup pine nuts or chopped walnuts

3 cloves garlic, smashed

Salt and black pepper

2 large tomatoes, chopped

1. Cook the pasta according to the package directions. Drain, saving ¼ cup of the pasta cooking water.

2. In a blender, combine the basil, oil, cheese, nuts, garlic, and salt and pepper to taste. Puree until blended and of the desired consistency.

3. In a large bowl, toss the pasta, reserved cooking water, and about 1 cup of the pesto. Toss in the tomatoes and season with salt and pepper to taste.

EveryGirl
TIP: This makes more than enough pesto for 1 pound of pasta. Reserve the leftovers to spread on sandwiches or add to soups and stews. The sauce will keep for a week in the refrigerator and in the freezer for a few months.

EveryGirl
TIP: Pesto is traditionally made with pine nuts. Sadly, they are expensive. Walnuts make a fine substitute.

Dolmades

MAKES ABOUT 20 DOLMADES

This recipe is diabetic-friendly and gluten-free!

This is a traditional Greek dish and one I can't live without. Filling grape leaves is a labor of love, so why not enlist the help of a loved one to make them? It's not hard, but it takes some time . . . time spent together.

1 tablespoon olive oil

1 small onion, chopped

¾ pound lean ground beef

½ cup cooked brown rice

¼ cup chopped fresh parsley

2 tablespoons chopped fresh mint

Zest from 1 lemon (about 1 tablespoon)

Salt and black pepper

1 jar (8 ounces) grape leaves

2 cups reduced-sodium chicken broth

2 egg yolks

¼ cup fresh lemon juice (from 2 lemons)

> **EveryGirl**
>
> **TIP:** You can serve these warm or at room temperature. I like to squeeze fresh lemon on top, and the lemon sauce is a wonderful creamy addition, but you could also serve the leaves without it.

1. Warm the oil in a large skillet with at least 2–inch sides over medium heat. Add the onion; cook for 6 minutes, stirring.

2. Add the beef; cook for 6 minutes, or until browned, stirring. Stir in the rice, parsley, mint, zest, and salt and pepper to taste.

3. Drain and blot the grape leaves dry with a paper towel. Line the bottom of a large Dutch oven or pot with some of the grape leaves.

4. Lay the remaining leaves out on the counter; stuff each with about 1 tablespoon of the filling. Roll up the leaves. Place the stuffed leaves in the pot, fitting them snugly in a single layer. Add the broth to barely cover the rolls. Bring to a boil; cover and let simmer for 30 minutes, or until the leaves are tender and the filling is hot.

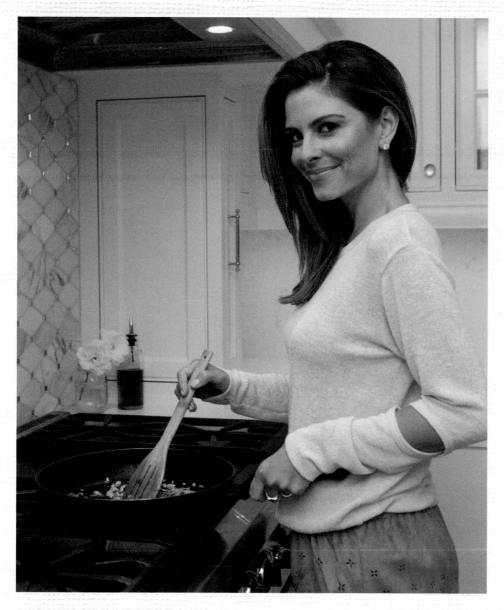

5. Using tongs, transfer the stuffed leaves to a large, shallow bowl. Pour the broth from the pot into a measuring cup.

6. In a large bowl, whisk the egg yolks and lemon juice until frothy. Slowly whisk the warm broth into the egg-juice mixture, a little at a time.

7. Pour this creamy lemon sauce over the grape leaves on a platter.

Chicken with Spring Vegetables

SERVES 3   This recipe is diabetic-friendly and gluten-free!

For a bigger meal, serve this beautifully bright green dish atop a bed of brown rice or your favorite grain, as seen here.

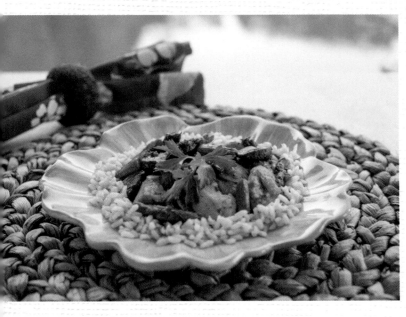

1 cup brown rice

3 tablespoons olive oil

2 boneless, skinless chicken breast halves, cut into 1-inch cubes

Salt and black pepper

1 cup reduced-sodium chicken broth

8 ounces asparagus, ends trimmed, thickly sliced on the diagonal

8 ounces white or cremini mushrooms, sliced

1 medium shallot or small onion, minced

1 tablespoon grated lemon zest

EveryGirl
TIP: Shallots are a milder form of onion. You can use a regular onion instead or omit the shallots altogether.

1. Bring the rice and 2½ cups water to a boil in a medium saucepan over high heat. Reduce the heat to low and simmer, covered, for about 45 minutes, or until the rice is tender and most of the liquid has been absorbed. Fluff with a fork.

2. Warm the oil in a large cast-iron or heavy skillet over medium-high heat.

3. Add the chicken, season with salt and pepper, and cook, stirring for 8 minutes, or until the chicken is lightly browned.

4. Add the broth, stirring to scrape up the browned bits at the bottom of the pan. Add the asparagus, mushrooms, shallot, and lemon zest; cover and cook for 5 minutes, stirring occasionally.

5. Uncover, cook for 2 minutes, or until the chicken is cooked through and the vegetables are tender-crisp. Serve with the rice.

Lemon Summer-Squash Bow Ties

SERVES 3 TO 4

If you use whole wheat pasta, this recipe is diabetic-friendly. **D** **GF**
Use gluten-free pasta and it becomes gluten-free, too!

Now that summer squash (zucchini and yellow squash) is available year-round, you can serve this easy dish any time of the year.

- ½ pound bow tie or penne pasta (regular, whole grain, or gluten-free)
- ¼ cup olive oil
- 2 medium or 4 small zucchini or yellow squash, shredded
- 3 cloves garlic, minced
- Zest of 1 lemon
- Salt and black pepper
- 3 tablespoons prepared or homemade basil pesto or chopped fresh parsley
- Grated Parmesan cheese, as desired

1. Cook the pasta according to the package directions. Drain, reserving ¼ cup of the cooking water.

2. Warm the oil in a large skillet over medium heat. Add the zucchini, garlic, and lemon zest; cook for 3 minutes, or until tender, stirring. Season with salt and pepper to taste.

3. In a large bowl, blend the pesto and reserved cooking water. Add the drained pasta and zucchini; toss to combine. Garnish the servings with cheese.

EveryGirl **TIP:** You want about 1 tablespoon of lemon zest here, but there is no need to actually measure it. Since you've got the grater out to shred the zucchini, use it to zest the lemon, too (no need to wash it).

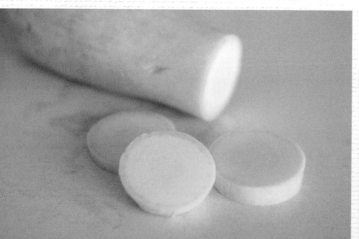

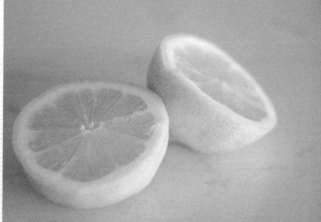

Simple-Roasted Salmon Fillets and Cherry Tomato Salad

SERVES 4

This recipe is diabetic-friendly and gluten-free!

Memorize this recipe for whenever you have to cook salmon. It's simple, straightforward, and utterly foolproof. Just remember to preheat the skillet before adding the salmon.

Salmon
2 tablespoons unsalted butter
2 tablespoons olive oil
4 salmon fillets, about 5 ounces each
2 tablespoons paprika
1 teaspoon granulated garlic
Salt and black pepper

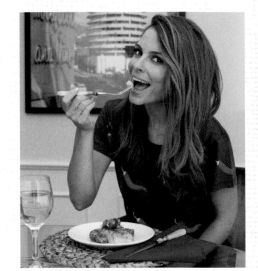

Salad
1 orange
1 pint cherry tomatoes, halved
½ cup chopped fresh parsley

1. Preheat the oven to 450°F.

2. For the salmon: Put the butter and oil in a large cast-iron or ovenproof skillet and place in the oven until the butter is melted and sizzling.

3. Season the salmon with the paprika, garlic, and salt and pepper to taste; add to the hot pan, skin side up. Place in the oven; roast for 5 minutes.

4. Using tongs, flip the fillets. Return to the oven; roast for 4 minutes, or until cooked to desired doneness.

5. For the salad: Using the smallest holes of a cheese grater, grate the peel from the orange into a bowl. Add the tomatoes and parsley. Serve over the salmon.

Greek Beef Stew

SERVES 6   Use 2 medium *red* potatoes instead of Yukon or other large potatoes and this is a **D** **GF** diabetic-friendly recipe. Either way, it's gluten-free!

This recipe was passed down to Mom from my grandfather in Greece; it's a family favorite.

3 tablespoons olive oil

1 pound chuck beef cubes

Salt and black pepper

2 Yukon Gold or large red potatoes, cubed

1 pound pearl onions, peeled but left whole

3 cloves garlic, minced

2 teaspoons minced fresh rosemary

1 can (14 ounces) tomato sauce

1 can (14 ounces) reduced-sodium beef broth

1. Warm 2 tablespoons of the oil in a large, heavy saucepan over medium-high heat. Add the beef and salt and pepper to taste, and cook for 5 minutes, turning until seared on all sides. Remove the beef to a bowl.

2. Add the remaining 1 tablespoon oil to the pan over medium heat. Add the potatoes, onions, garlic, rosemary, tomato sauce, beef broth, and meat and bring to a simmer. Reduce the heat to low, partially cover, and cook for 40 minutes, or until the meat is tender and the vegetables are cooked through.

EveryGirl

TIP: Look for beef labeled "Beef for Stew" at your butcher shop or market.

EveryGirl

TIP: If you can't find, or can't be bothered with peeling, the pearl onions, just dice a large onion and use that instead.

Melted Baked Ziti with Charred Cauliflower

SERVES 6

Serve this simple grown-up mac and cheese with a crisp green salad. Alter the cheese to suit your taste.

3 tablespoons olive oil, plus extra for the pan

¾ pound ziti or other tube pasta (regular, whole-wheat, or rice)

1 large head cauliflower, core removed and florets quartered or halved if small

2 cloves garlic, chopped

1 teaspoon chopped fresh thyme

1 teaspoon lemon zest (from 1 lemon)

¾ cup (about 6 ounces) shredded Gruyère or Swiss cheese

Salt and black pepper

½ cup grated Parmesan or Romano cheese

1. Preheat the oven to 400°F. Lightly oil a 9 x 13-inch baking dish.

2. Cook the pasta according to the package directions, but drain a few minutes before completely cooked, while still al dente.

3. Warm the 3 tablespoons oil in a large, heavy skillet over medium-high heat. Add the cauliflower and cook for 3 minutes, until spotty brown on one side. Shake the pan to flip the florets, and brown the other side. Transfer the cauliflower to the prepared baking dish.

4. Add the garlic to the skillet; cook for 30 seconds, stirring. Transfer to the baking dish.

5. Add the drained pasta, the thyme, lemon zest, and Gruyère to the cauliflower in the baking dish, season with salt and pepper to taste, and stir to combine. Sprinkle evenly with the Parmesan. Bake, uncovered, for 20 minutes, or until the top is crisp and golden.

Family-Style Crispy Chicken Tenders with Rice and Beans

SERVES 4

Adding just a couple of spices turns a can of beans into a delicious side dish!

1 pound chicken tenders

Salt and black pepper

½ cup all-purpose flour

2 large eggs

1 cup panko or regular bread crumbs

1 cup grated Parmesan cheese

Vegetable oil, for frying

1 can (15 ounces) black beans, drained and rinsed

2 teaspoons ground cumin

½ teaspoon chili powder

2 cups cooked brown or white rice

1. Season the chicken tenders with salt and pepper to taste. Set up three shallow bowls for dipping; one bowl with the flour, one with the beaten eggs, and one with a combination of the panko and Parmesan.

2. Dip each tender in the flour, then the eggs, then the panko-cheese mixture, coating both sides completely.

3. Add the vegetable oil to about ½ inch up the sides of a large, heavy skillet over high heat. Cook the tenders for about 3 minutes per side, or until evenly browned and cooked through. Using tongs, remove to a paper towel–lined plate.

4. Meanwhile, warm the beans, cumin, and chili powder, and season with salt and pepper to taste in a small saucepan over low heat. Mound ½ cup of the warm rice onto a serving platter. Top with the warm beans and chicken.

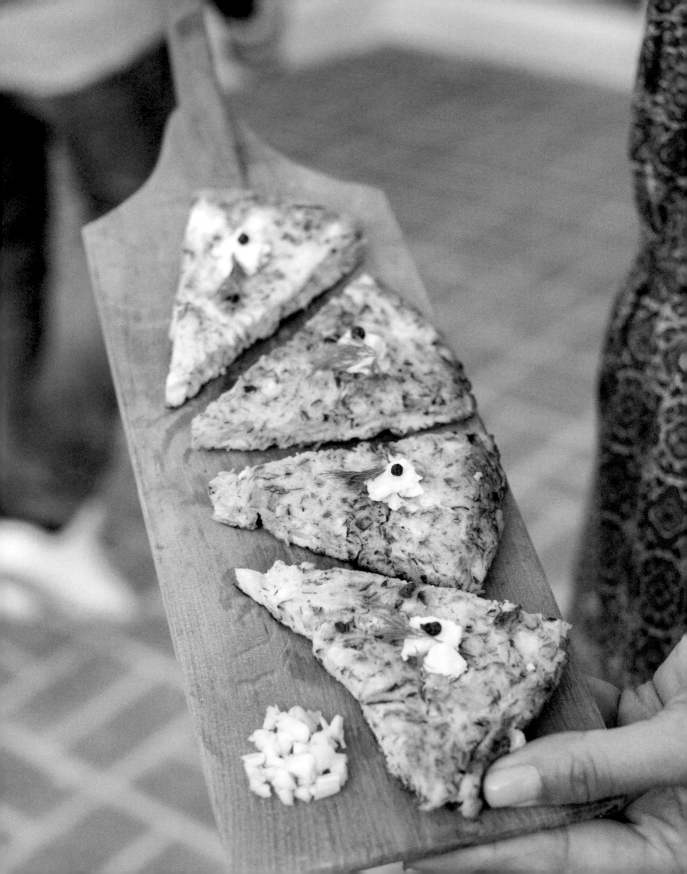

Zucchini and Feta Cheese Frittata

SERVES 2   This recipe is diabetic-friendly and gluten-free!

Zucchini and dill are a classic flavor combination. If you don't care for dill, feel free to substitute thyme, parsley, or basil. Or skip the herbs altogether.

2 tablespoons olive oil

1 large zucchini, grated (about 2 cups)

2 cloves garlic, minced

4 large eggs

Salt and black pepper

¼ cup crumbled feta cheese (use goat cheese, if you prefer)

2 tablespoons chopped fresh dill

1. Warm 1 tablespoon of the oil in an 8-inch nonstick skillet over medium heat. Add the zucchini; cook 4 minutes, or until the zucchini softens, stirring. Add the garlic; cook for 30 seconds, stirring.

2. In a large bowl, beat the eggs and salt and pepper to taste. Stir in the zucchini mixture, cheese, and dill.

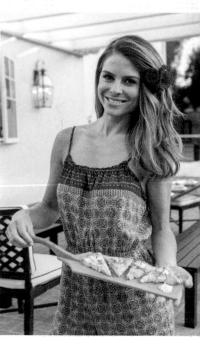

3. Wipe out the skillet with a paper towel and place over medium-high heat. Warm the remaining 1 tablespoon oil. Pour the egg mixture into the hot pan. Stir to distribute evenly. During the first few minutes of cooking, tilt the pan slightly while lifting up the edges of the frittata with a spatula to let the uncooked eggs run underneath.

4. Reduce the heat to low; cover and cook for a few minutes, until the top of the frittata is just set, shaking the pan gently a few times.

5. Run a spatula around the edges of the pan to loosen the frittata from the pan. Slide the frittata onto a cutting board. Flip the frittata so that the top of the frittata lands in the skillet. Place the pan over low heat; cook a few minutes, until the bottom of the frittata is golden. Slide from the pan onto a platter.

Warm Sweet Potato Salad with Kale and Brown Rice

SERVES 4

This recipe is diabetic-friendly and gluten-free!

You can use any grain in this salad. Just remember, cooking times vary with the type of grain used.

2 sweet potatoes (1½ pounds), unpeeled, cut into 1-inch chunks

2 tablespoons olive oil

Salt and black pepper

½ cup brown rice

1 large onion, thinly sliced

3 tablespoons apple cider vinegar

2 tablespoons maple syrup

½ bunch (about 6 ounces) kale, stems removed and leaves coarsely chopped

1. Preheat the oven to 375°F.

2. Spread the sweet potatoes on a foil-lined baking sheet. Drizzle with 1 tablespoon of the oil; sprinkle with salt and pepper. Roast for 20 to 25 minutes, until tender, stirring the potatoes during cooking.

3. Meanwhile, cook the rice according to the package directions until tender but chewy. Transfer to a large serving bowl.

4. Warm the remaining 1 tablespoon oil in a medium saucepan over low heat. Cook the onion for 15 minutes, or until lightly browned, stirring often.

5. Add the vinegar and syrup; cook for 5 minutes, stirring.

6. Stir in the kale and cook for 5 minutes, until wilted, stirring.

7. Add the potatoes and slightly mash to a chunky consistency. Fold the mixture into the rice in the bowl.

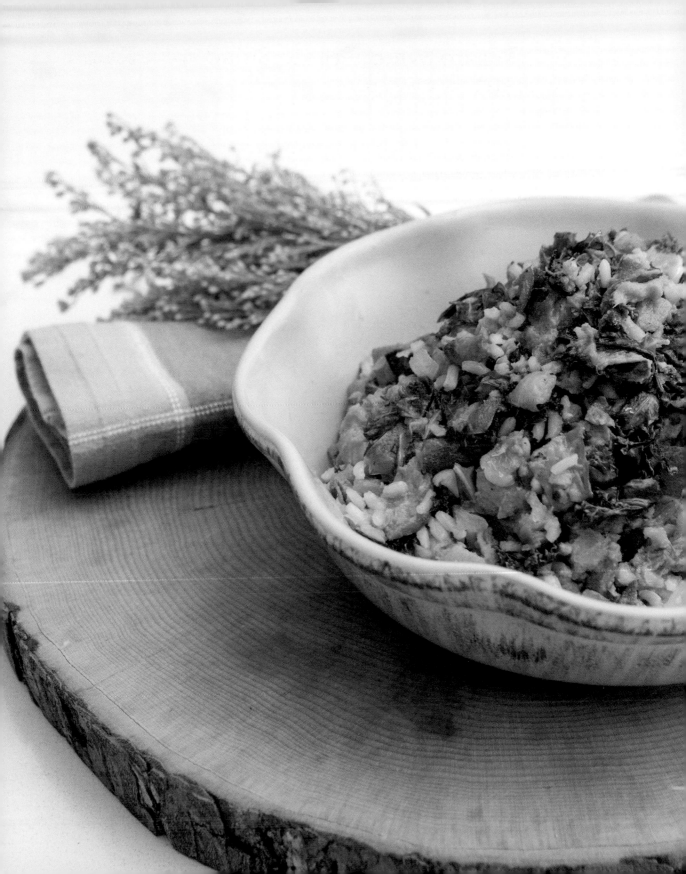

Potato-Onion Stew

SERVES 4

Use this recipe as a starting point. Want it meatier? Cook a few strips of bacon and crumble them into the soup at the end. Greener? Stir in some chopped spinach or kale at the end.

4 tablespoons olive oil

1 large onion, chopped

2 cloves garlic, minced

3 russet potatoes, peeled and cut into small dice

1 fresh rosemary sprig

Salt and black pepper

4 cups (32 ounces) reduced-sodium chicken broth

Grated Parmesan cheese, as desired

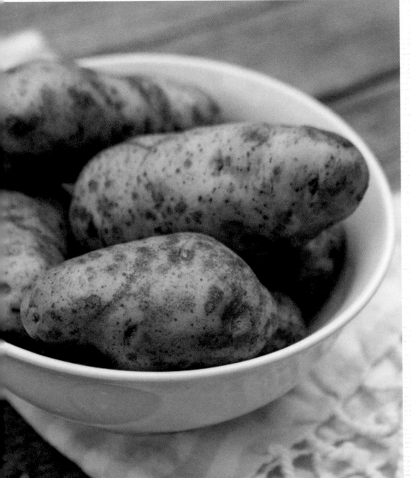

1. Warm the oil in a large soup pot or Dutch oven over medium-low heat. Add the onion and cook for 5 minutes, stirring.

2. Add the garlic; cook for 30 seconds, stirring. Add the potatoes and rosemary, and salt and pepper to taste, stirring.

3. Add the broth; increase the heat and bring to a simmer. Reduce the heat; simmer for 30 minutes, or until the potatoes are tender.

4. Remove the rosemary sprig. Garnish with the Parmesan.

Baked Potato Frittata

SERVES 2

One of my personal favorites—goes with almost everything!

    2 tablespoons olive oil
    1 large or 2 small yellow potatoes, such as Yukon Gold, halved and
        thinly sliced
    ½ red bell pepper, thinly sliced
    ½ small red onion, thinly sliced
    4 large eggs
    ½ cup (2 ounces) crumbled feta cheese
    2 tablespoons chopped fresh parsley
    ½ teaspoon crushed red pepper, or to taste
    Salt and black pepper

1. Preheat the oven to 350°F.

2. Warm the oil in a medium, nonstick, ovenproof skillet over medium heat. Add the potatoes, red bell pepper, and onion; cook for 8 minutes, or until the potatoes are golden, stirring often.

3. In a medium bowl, whisk the eggs, feta, parsley, crushed red pepper, and salt and black pepper to taste. Pour over the mixture in the skillet; stir gently to distribute evenly.

4. Place in the oven and bake for 25 minutes, or until the frittata is just firm to the touch.

EveryGirl
TIP: Use a nonstick skillet for frittatas and omelets so they'll slide right out of the pan. If you don't have nonstick, just serve the meal out of the skillet—it will still be delicious! Since this frittata spends some time in the oven, make sure your skillet has an oven-safe handle.

Linguine with Lemon-Garlic Shrimp

SERVES 4

This one is a classic made better for all the lemony goodness!

EveryGirl

TIP: Save time by purchasing shrimp that have already been peeled and deveined.

EveryGirl

TIP: Remember to zest the lemon before juicing it. Use the smallest holes on a cheese grater.

12 ounces linguine (regular, whole-wheat, or rice)

3 tablespoons olive oil

4 cloves garlic, minced

¼ to ½ teaspoon red pepper flakes, as desired

1 pound medium shrimp, peeled and deveined

1 lemon, zested and juiced

Salt

3 tablespoons butter, cut into chunks

½ cup chopped fresh parsley

1. Cook the pasta according to the package directions; drain.

2. Warm the oil in a large skillet over medium-low heat. Add the garlic and pepper flakes and cook for 20 seconds, stirring.

3. Add the shrimp in an even layer; sprinkle with the lemon zest and salt and cook for 1 minute. Turn the shrimp and cook for 2 minutes, stirring.

4. Remove the skillet from the heat; stir in the butter, lemon juice, and parsley. Toss in the hot pasta until coated.

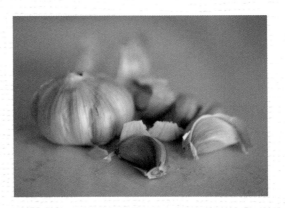

Shrimp, Red Pepper, and Swiss Chard Sauté over Rice

SERVES 4   Use brown rice and this recipe is diabetic-friendly. Either way it's gluten-free!

Simply delicious! I've really become a big fan of Swiss chard. I grow it in my garden. Another impressive meal that's easy to make.

2 tablespoons olive oil

1 medium red onion, thinly sliced

1 red bell pepper, cut into thin slices

2 cloves garlic, minced

1 small bunch Swiss chard (about 8 ounces), trimmed and coarsely chopped

1 pound medium shrimp, peeled and deveined

Salt and black pepper

2 cups cooked brown rice

1. Warm the oil in a large saucepan over medium heat. Add the onion, red pepper, and garlic; cook for 5 minutes, stirring.

2. Stir in the chard and shrimp; cook for 5 minutes, or until the shrimp is cooked through and the chard is wilted, stirring.

3. Season with salt and pepper to taste. Serve over the rice.

EveryGirl

TIP: To prep the chard, slice off the stems, then remove the thick rib from the middle of the leaf. Spinach is a fine, and easy-to-prep, substitute.

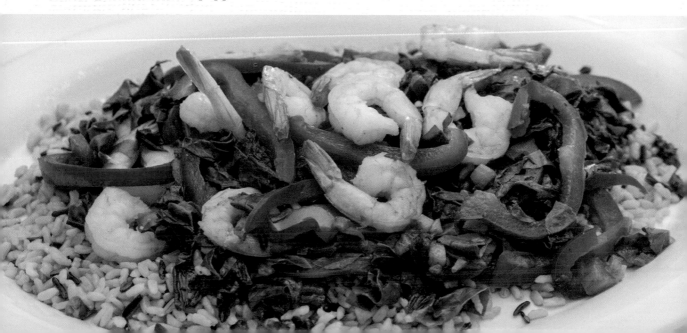

Over-Loaded Stuffed Potatoes

SERVES 4

Vegetarian? Just omit the ground beef. But do try this delicious self-contained meal!

2 large russet potatoes

2 teaspoons olive oil

8 ounces ground beef

1 medium tomato, chopped

2 scallions, thinly sliced

Salt and black pepper

½ cup shredded Cheddar cheese, or 4 ounces Velveeta cheese, cubed

½ cup reduced-fat sour cream, as desired

EveryGirl

TIP: Potato baking times will vary depending on the size of your spuds. You want them to be cooked through.

1. Preheat the oven to 375°F.

2. Rub the outside of the potatoes with the oil. Bake for 50 minutes, or until softened. Slice horizontally and scoop out the flesh of the potatoes; reserve the potato shells.

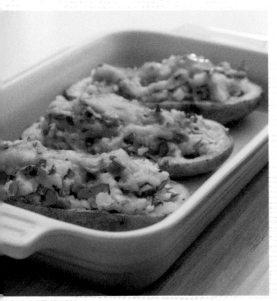

3. Place the flesh in a bowl and mash. Maintain the oven temperature.

4. Meanwhile, cook the beef in a heavy skillet over medium heat until browned.

5. Add the tomato, scallions, mashed potatoes, and salt and pepper to taste. Cook for 1 minute.

6. Spoon the mixture into the potato shells; sprinkle evenly with the cheese.

7. Place on a baking sheet and bake for 15 minutes, or until the cheese is melted.

8. Top with the sour cream if using.

Black-Eyed Pea and Collard Greens Soup

SERVES 6 TO 8   This recipe is diabetic-friendly and gluten-free!

In my house, we eat a lot of beans! This recipe incorporates our love of black-eyed peas with a Southern influence.

  2 cups (about 1 pound) dried black-eyed peas
  2 tablespoons olive oil
  4 carrots, peeled and thinly sliced
  1 stalk celery, sliced
  1 large onion, diced
  2 cloves garlic, minced
  4 cups (32 ounces) reduced-sodium chicken or vegetable broth
  1 can (8 ounces) tomato sauce
  1 small bunch collard greens (about 8 ounces), tough stems and ribs
    removed, leaves thinly sliced
  1 tablespoon red wine vinegar
  Salt and black pepper
  Cayenne pepper

EveryGirl

TIP: This recipe makes 9 cups of hearty, thick soup. If you want a soupier soup, just add more water during the cooking time. Leftovers will keep for several days in the refrigerator and make a great bring-to-work lunch.

1. In a large bowl, cover the peas with water by at least 3 inches and let soak overnight. Drain and rinse well.

2. Warm the oil in a large saucepan over medium heat. Add the carrots, celery, onion, and garlic; cook for 6 minutes, or until the onion is softened, stirring.

3. Add the drained peas, broth, tomato sauce, and 3 cups water; bring to a simmer. Reduce the heat and simmer, partially covered, for 40 minutes, or until the peas are tender. Add water as needed if the soup becomes too dry.

4. Add the collard greens; cook for 15 minutes, or until the greens are wilted.

5. Stir in the vinegar. Season with salt, pepper, and cayenne to taste.

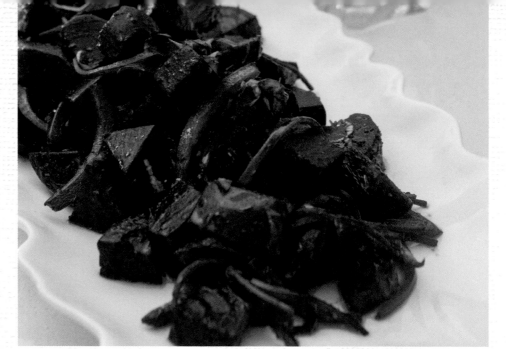

Beet Salad

SERVES 4   This recipe is diabetic-friendly and gluten-free! **D** **GF**

I have always disliked beets, but I love this salad!!! And now, I'm a big fan of beets because of it.

4 large beets, washed and unpeeled
Salt
1 red onion, sliced
3 tablespoons olive oil
2 tablespoons rice-wine, apple-cider, or white-wine vinegar
1 teaspoon Italian spice blend
2 tablespoons sliced fresh basil

1. In a medium saucepan, cover the beets with water and season with salt. Bring to a boil over high heat. Boil until tender. Drain and rinse with cold water. Peel and dice the beets.

2. In a large bowl, combine the diced beets with the red onion, olive oil, vinegar, spice blend, and basil. Toss to coat.

Chicken and Broccoli Rigatoni

SERVES 4

The reserved pasta cooking water, along with the cheese and garlic oil, make the sauce for this savory dish.

- ½ pound rigatoni or other medium pasta (regular, whole-wheat, or rice)
- ⅓ cup olive oil
- 1 pound boneless, skinless chicken breast halves, thinly sliced
- Salt and black pepper
- 5 cloves garlic, peeled and smashed
- ¼ teaspoon red pepper flakes
- 2 stalks broccoli, florets sliced, stalks peeled and thinly sliced
- ¾ cup grated Parmesan cheese

1. Cook the pasta according to the package directions; before draining, put aside ¼ cup cooking water for later. Drain the rest of the water from the pasta.

2. Warm the oil in a medium skillet over medium heat. Season the chicken with salt and pepper to taste; add to the skillet, along with the garlic and red pepper flakes. Cook, stirring, until the garlic turns golden.

3. Using a slotted spoon, remove the garlic cloves from the pan and discard.

4. Add the broccoli to the skillet; cook for 5 minutes, or until tender-crisp.

5. Add the drained pasta; toss to coat, adding pasta water and the cheese to make a thin sauce. Season to taste with salt and pepper.

EveryGirl
TIP: There's no need to discard the broccoli stalks. Just chop off the woody ends and thinly slice the rest of the stalk.

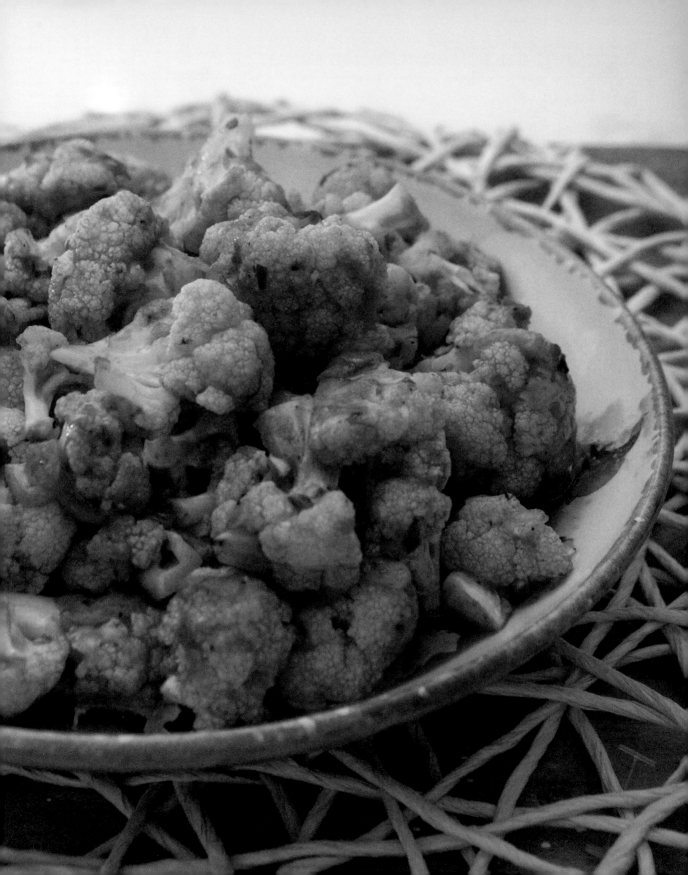

Simple Cauliflower Sauté

SERVES 4   This recipe is diabetic-friendly and gluten-free! **D** **GF**

Bay leaf adds a subtle, almost tea-like flavor to a dish. If you don't have any on hand, feel free to leave it out.

½ cup olive oil
2 large onions, diced
1 head cauliflower, chopped
1 can (7 ounces) tomato sauce
¼ cup chopped fresh parsley
¼ cup water (or vegetable broth)
1 sprinkle of crushed red pepper flakes
1 bay leaf
Salt and black pepper

1. Warm the oil in a large skillet over medium heat. Add the onions, and cook for 10 minutes, or until caramelized.

2. Add the cauliflower; cook for 2 minutes, stirring.

3. Add the sauce; cook for 2 minutes.

4. Stir in the parsley, water, crushed red pepper flakes, bay leaf, and salt and black pepper to taste. Cook for 10 minutes, or until the cauliflower is tender. Remove the bay leaf before serving.

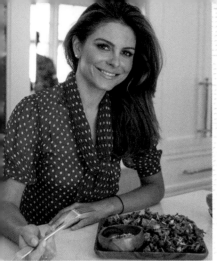

Autumn Kale Salad with Apple and Cider Vinaigrette

SERVES 6 TO 8

If you skip the apple juice and cranberries, this recipe is diabetic-friendly!

Unlike most greens, the flavor of kale improves when you dress the leaves in advance. So go ahead and dress the salad, then prep your add-ins. Got leftovers? Don't throw them out—the salad will keep in the fridge for tomorrow's lunch.

3 tablespoons extra-virgin olive oil

1 tablespoon apple cider vinegar

1 tablespoon apple cider or apple juice

Salt and black pepper

1 large bunch (12 ounces to 1 pound) kale, stems removed and leaves coarsely chopped

1 large tart apple, such as Honey Crisp or Gala, diced

½ cup sweetened dried cranberries

½ cup sliced almonds

½ cup finely shredded Romano or Parmesan cheese

1. In a large serving bowl, whisk the oil, vinegar, apple cider, and salt and pepper to taste. Add the kale, toss with your hands, and massage the dressing into the leaves.

2. Add the apple, cranberries, almonds, and cheese; toss to coat.

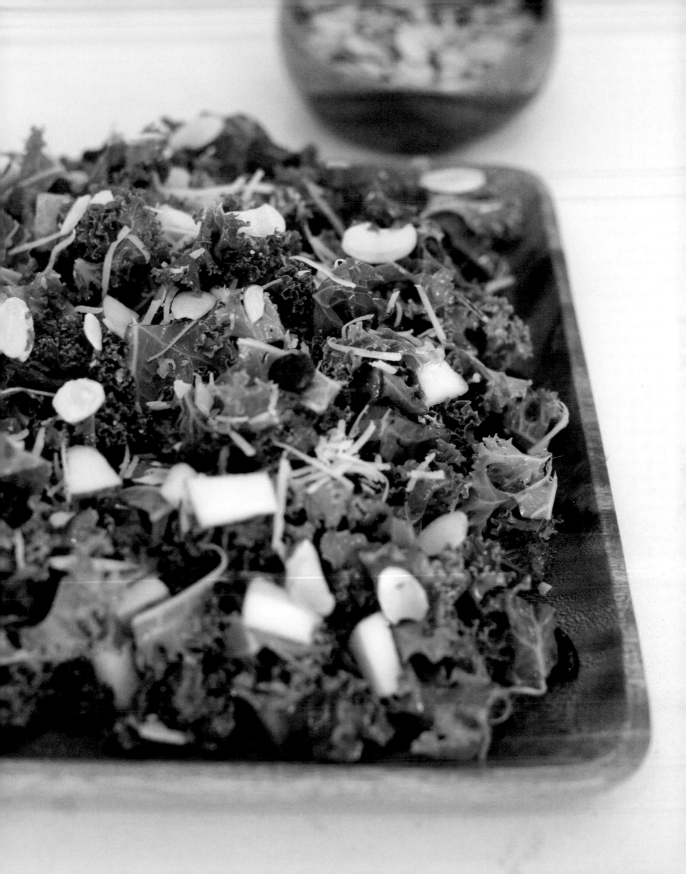

Cucumber and Yogurt Soup

SERVES 6   This recipe is diabetic-friendly and gluten-free!

This soup is served cold, so it makes a great make-ahead dish.

6 cucumbers, peeled and diced

3 cups plain Greek yogurt

¼ cup chopped fresh parsley

1 clove garlic, minced

1. Combine the cucumbers, yogurt, parsley, and garlic in a food processor; puree until smooth.

2. Refrigerate until ready to serve.

I like the nutritional benefits of the cucumber peel so I tend to take a fork down the sides and keep the rest of the peel intact. Do as you like!

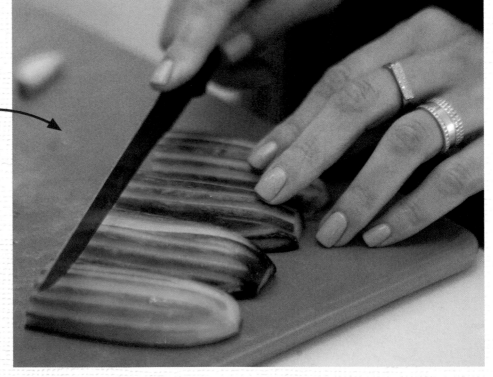

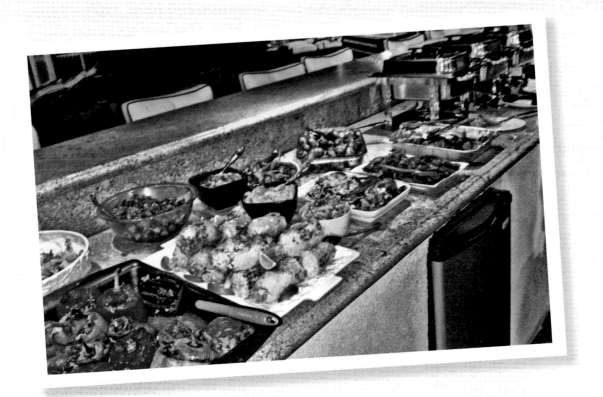

EveryGirl CELEBRITY COOKING MOMENT

Nia Vardalos introduced me to my first potluck "cook off" competition. She hosted one at her house, inviting all her friends, including the equally lovely and talented Melina Kanakaredes, fellow Greek, and star of *CSI: New York*. After we feasted on some of the most amazing dishes, we were given ballots to vote and comment on our favorites. It was so much fun and far more festive than a simple dinner party. I was hooked on the concept from then on and learned some of the most incredible recipes, too.

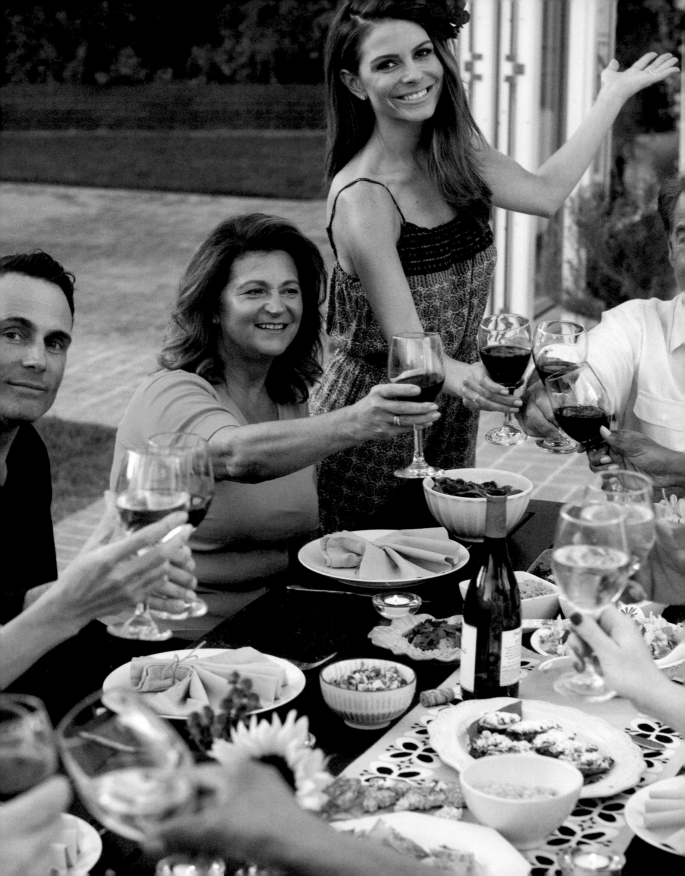

EveryGirl

ENTERTAINS

I love entertaining! Maybe that's why I'm a TV host. I honestly love it so much that when I entertain, I always try to outdo myself. My birthday bashes are always pretty epic, but I also love smaller affairs such as hosting girls' dinners. Sometimes we'll do potlucks, where all my friends bring their favorite dishes. FYI, potlucks make it way easier to host dinner parties especially during busy workweeks. I've also found that a lot of my girlfriends love the excuse to cook for more than just themselves. The potluck becomes something they get excited about as an opportunity to show off their cooking powers. There are a few other things I've learned along the way in terms of entertaining.

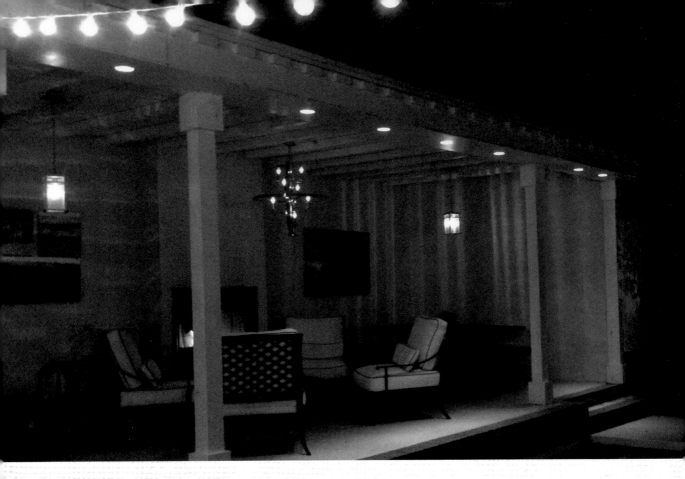

Lighting

Always set the mood. If it's a dinner party, be sure to dim your lights and light some candles. Before my guests arrive, I spend a good amount of time running around my house and turning on key indoor and outdoor lights. Lighting is everything!

Music

Create a dinner party playlist or use a service like Spotify. My favorite dinner party music is good old Frank Sinatra and Tony Bennett. If we want the party to turn into a dance party, then I have a great dance mix of classics combined with Top 40 hits.

Drinks

Try to greet guests with drinks. If that's too much, create a table setting with a bottle each of white and red wine, a basic alcohol like vodka, mixers, some sparkling water or a pitcher of water, chopped lemons and limes, ice, and glasses on a tray. It looks fancy, doesn't require much effort, and enables guests to help themselves.

Appetizers

It's a nice idea to have food for people to nibble on before the big meal. Be sure to set some finger food out on the table a few minutes before guests arrive. Some good go-to cheats are pre-made cheese platters and veggie platters. Also see my appetizer ideas starting on page 141.

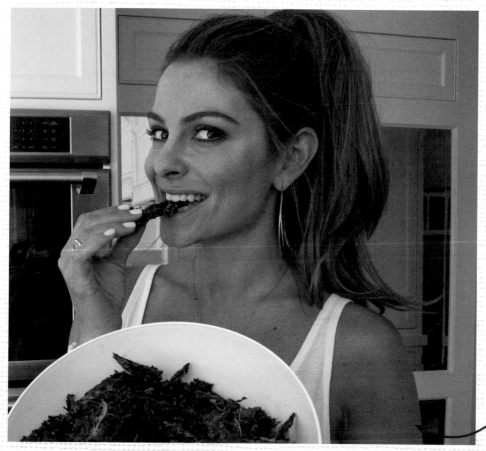

Kale chips are easy and delicious!

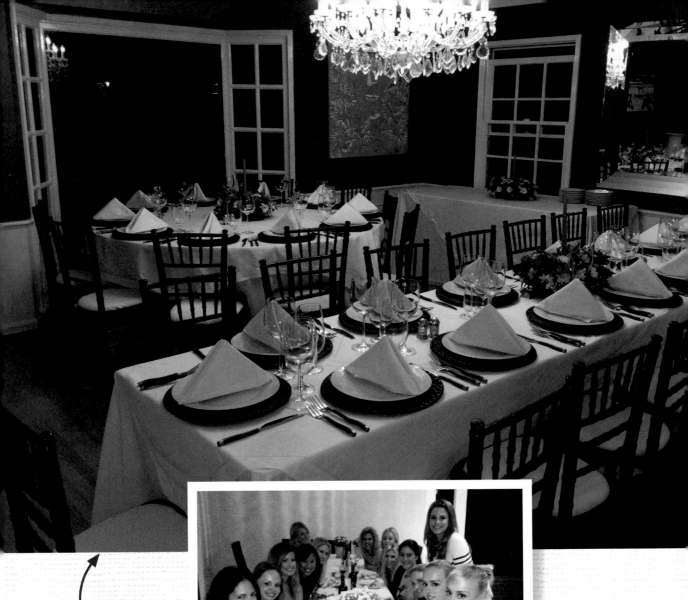

My Thanksgiving day dinner setup. I rent extra chairs and place settings so everyone can sit together and things match.

One of my girls' night potluck dinners.

Meal

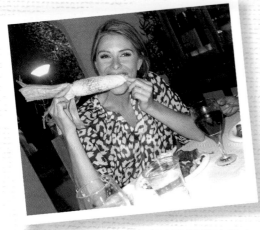

In terms of the meal, I always make more than enough. There's nothing worse than having guests be afraid that there isn't enough for everyone when serving themselves! You can enjoy the leftovers tomorrow. Keven calls this cooking "the Italian way," though it sure is the Greek way, too!

And remember to ask your guests if they have any dietary restrictions and be mindful of having items on your menu that will work for everyone. Since my dad is diabetic, cousins, uncles, and aunts who hosted us always took that into consideration. Others may keep kosher, have gluten allergies, or be vegan or vegetarian. It's always smart to ask nowadays.

When you have your menu, think about what you can prep ahead of time to make the actual evening easier on you. I used to spend the entire night in the kitchen and miss out on the entertaining part! Now I try to do as much prep as I can before guests arrive—chopping potatoes and keeping them in water in the fridge or making dips and dressings ahead of time—so I can enjoy our guests and the evening.

And why not print out your menu? Rather than telling everyone what each item will be, print the full menu and frame it. I do this at the holidays all the time. For a smaller dinner party, I handwrite the name of each item on a folded piece of paper and set it in front of the item. It's those little touches that impress people.

EveryGirl
TIP: Check out my other *EveryGirl's Guide* books for go-to entertaining recipes like my *EveryGirl Nachos*, *Black Bean–Mango Salad*, and *Stuffed Eggplant with Feta and Ricotta Cheese*—all big hits!

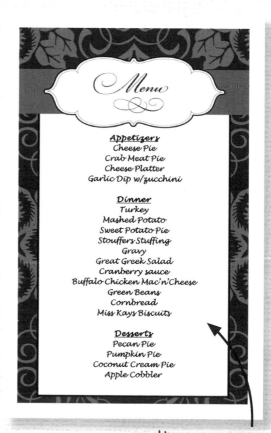

Menu

Appetizers
Cheese Pie
Crab Meat Pie
Cheese Platter
Garlic Dip w/zucchini

Dinner
Turkey
Mashed Potato
Sweet Potato Pie
Stouffers Stuffing
Gravy
Great Greek Salad
Cranberry sauce
Buffalo Chicken Mac'n'Cheese
Green Beans
Cornbread
Miss Kays Biscuits

Desserts
Pecan Pie
Pumpkin Pie
Coconut Cream Pie
Apple Cobbler

My Thanksgiving menu!

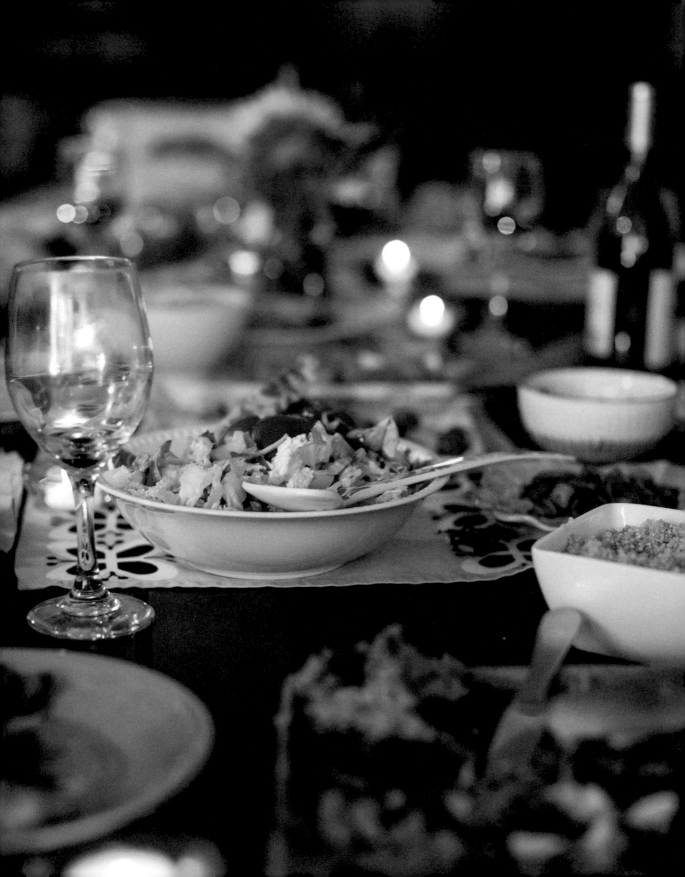

Details

If your dinner party is outside, place a few sweatshirts or throw blankets in a box so guests can feel free to grab one if it gets chilly.

For plates and silverware, I've done both real and plastic. For a super-fancy, I-gotta-impress-the-bosses kind of dinner, I go with real. If it's my friends and I have an early day the next day, I go with a finer plastic to make cleanup easy. Most people don't want to watch you slave over the sink, anyhow. For that reason, they want you to use plastic, too.

EveryGirl Splurges

Let's face it, everyone has a splurge food. I don't know about you, but I can't imagine a life where I could *never* have a chocolate chip cookie. You'll notice most of my splurge items are listed in this chapter. Here's why. Generally, you will be making these dishes when you are entertaining, which won't be every day. And when you entertain, you're entitled to enjoy yourself.

The beauty of the 75%/25% plan is that you never feel deprived. No food is forbidden. The key to a long, healthy life is moderation. Be most mindful of portion sizes—aim for balance, not perfection.

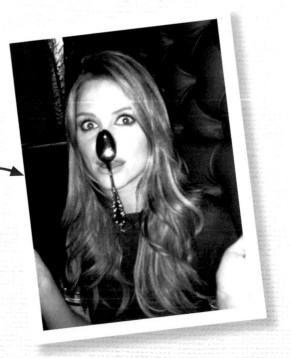

My dog Winnie is a lush! Remember to keep alcohol away from those under 21!

If your party needs an infusion of fun, see if you can do this with your guests. It always gets people laughing and talking and it's competitive in a fun way.

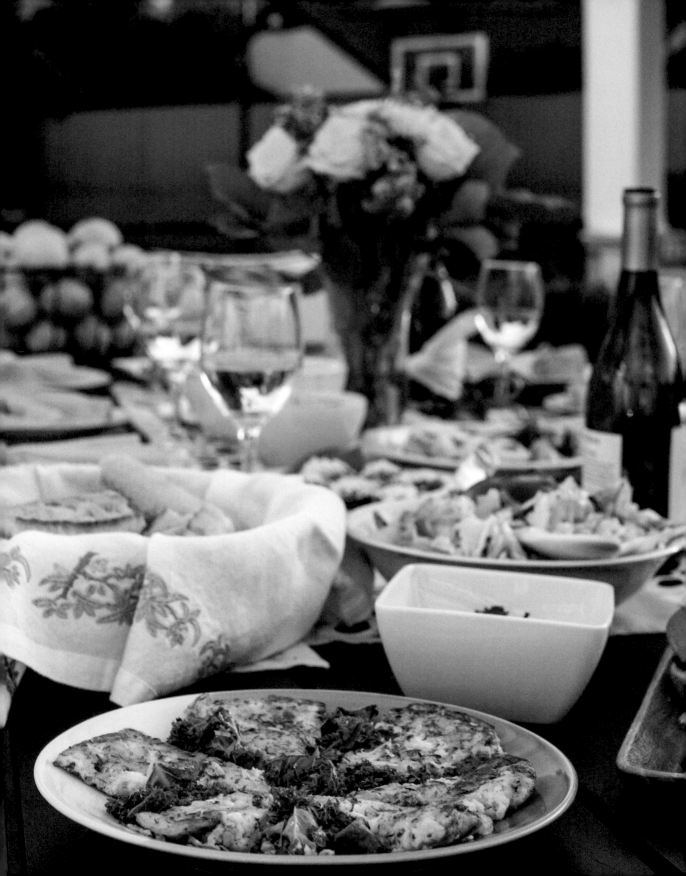

EveryGirl ENTERTAINS

Appetizers

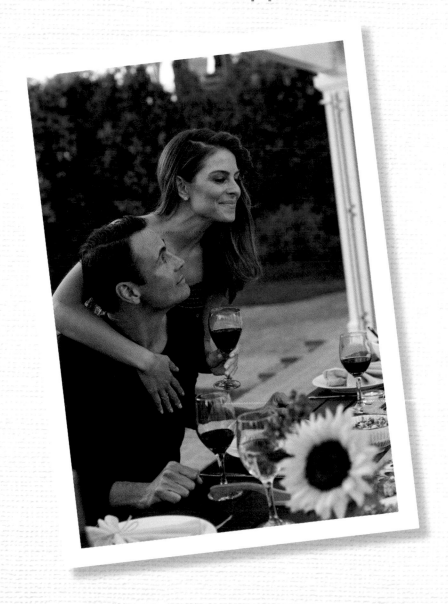

Roasted Sweet Potato Fries with Maple Hummus Dipping Sauce

SERVES 4

You can make these as spicy as you want by upping (or omitting) the cayenne pepper. You can also forgo the dip and serve with ketchup. Your guests are going to love them!

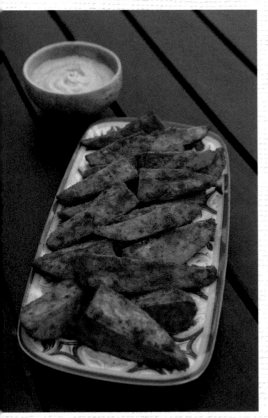

Sweet Potato Fries

2 pounds sweet potatoes (about 2 large)

2 tablespoons cornstarch

½ teaspoon garlic powder

1 teaspoon paprika

¼ teaspoon cayenne pepper, or to taste

Salt and black pepper

2 tablespoons olive oil

Maple Hummus Dipping Sauce

½ cup prepared or homemade hummus

1 tablespoon maple syrup

1. Preheat the oven to 400°F. Line two rimmed baking sheets with parchment paper. Cut the sweet potatoes into quarters, then into ½-inch-wide wedges.

2. In a large bowl, combine the cornstarch, garlic powder, paprika, cayenne, and salt and pepper to taste. Add the potato wedges; toss to coat. Drizzle with the oil; toss again. Spread the potatoes out onto the prepared baking sheets. Bake for 15 minutes, or until brown and crisp; flip the wedges and cook for 15 minutes, until the other side is crisp.

3. Meanwhile, make the dipping sauce. In a small bowl, stir together the hummus and maple syrup. Serve with the hot fries.

Sesame Hummus with Pita Crisps

MAKES ABOUT 1½ CUPS

The fresh parsley in this recipe whips up a lovely light-green dip—if you prefer the more traditional brown hummus, omit the herb. You could also experiment with another herb, like dill or basil.

  1 can (16 ounces) chickpeas, drained and rinsed
  Juice from 2 lemons (about ¼ cup)
  ¼ cup sesame oil
  ¼ cup chopped fresh parsley
  Salt, black pepper, and crushed red pepper, to taste
  2 to 3 tablespoons water
  Whole-wheat pita chips

Place all the ingredients except the water and chips in a food processor; puree until creamy. The mixture may still look grainy, so slowly add water as needed until the mixture looks creamy and light. Store, tightly covered, in the refrigerator. Serve cool or at room temperature with the pita chips.

EveryGirl
TIP: There are two different kinds of sesame oil at your market. The dark (or Asian) sesame oil is too intense for this recipe. Use the lighter, cooking sesame oil here.

Zucchini Toasts

MAKES ABOUT 12 TOASTS

Be careful with this one; if you make too many, people will eat so many of these and miss dinner! They are that good! Add crushed red pepper flakes if you want an extra little kick.

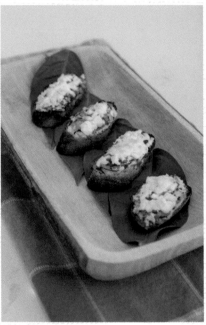

EveryGirl

TIP: Remember, broilers do their work quickly, so keep an eye on the toasts to make sure they don't burn. Set an alarm on your phone; that's what I do!

EveryGirl

TIP: The easiest method for drizzling oil is to place your index finger so that it covers most of the spout of the oil bottle. Tilt the bottle over the bread so just a thin stream runs past your finger and onto the bread.

2 teaspoons olive oil, plus additional for the bread

1 large zucchini, shredded

2 cloves garlic, minced

1 teaspoon minced fresh rosemary

2 tablespoons lemon zest (from 1 lemon)

Salt and black pepper

1 baguette, gluten-free if desired, cut into slices

½ cup part-skim ricotta cheese

½ cup (2 ounces) crumbled feta cheese

1. Preheat the broiler. Warm the 2 teaspoons oil in a large nonstick skillet over medium heat. Add the zucchini and garlic; cook for 3 minutes, stirring. Stir in the rosemary, lemon zest, and salt and pepper to taste.

2. Drizzle the cut sides of the baguette lightly with oil; broil until golden. Spread the ricotta on the toasts and top with the zucchini mixture. Top with the feta; broil until the cheese is bubbling.

Eggplant-Feta Mash

MAKES 1½ CUPS   This recipe is diabetic friendly and gluten-free!

Serve this savory side dish with hunks of bread for scooping. Celery and cucumber are great dipping alternatives.

1 large eggplant
1 clove garlic, minced
1 tablespoon olive oil
2 tablespoons crumbled feta cheese
2 tablespoons chopped fresh parsley
½ teaspoon chopped fresh oregano
Salt

1. Preheat the oven to 425°F.

2. Line a rimmed baking sheet with foil. Place the whole eggplant on the baking sheet; roast for 45 minutes to 1 hour, until soft when squeezed.

3. Let cool slightly; peel and coarsely chop.

4. Transfer to a medium bowl; add the garlic, oil, cheese, parsley, oregano, and salt to taste; mash to the desired chunkiness.

5. Serve warm.

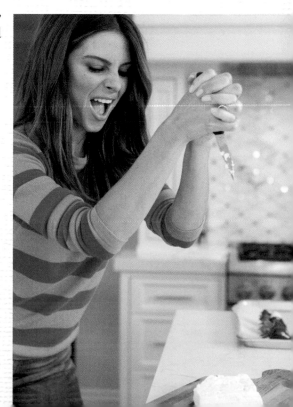

Tammie's Kale Chips

MAKES ABOUT 6 CHIPS PER LEAF   This recipe is diabetic-friendly and gluten-free! **D** **GF**

My friend Tammie makes amazing kale chips, and this is her recipe. I love to make a big batch to eat while watching movies instead of popcorn. Anyone who looks at me with that "I could never replace popcorn" look always takes it back once they try the kale chips! It's pretty genius!

EveryGirl

TIP: They are great little appetizers, too, instead of chips.

Curly kale
Olive oil
Salt

1. Preheat the oven to 325°F.

2. Take a few stalks of kale, wash, and dry. Starting at the bottom, gently tear off the leaves; kale grows in natural sections, so just pull it apart right where it separates, and place it in a bowl.

3. Pour a few teaspoons of olive oil over the kale and lightly coat all the leaves. Make sure each leaf is nicely covered with oil by giving the leaves a little massage to ensure full coverage.

4. Spread the leaves in a single layer on a sheet pan, and sprinkle with a little salt. For an added twist, use garlic salt or even salt-free seasoning.

5. Bake for 10 to 17 minutes, until crisp. Larger leaves take a little longer; smaller ones will cook faster. Keep an eye on them. Don't let them brown. Browned kale tastes bitter.

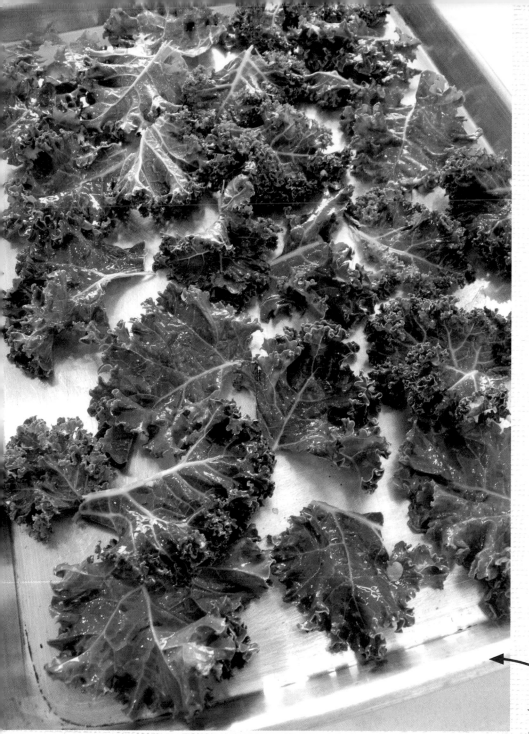

EveryGirl

TIP: Be sure to use curly kale; the flat-leaf kale doesn't crisp up enough to get that good crunch.

EveryGirl

TIP: Be careful with the salt; it's easy to overdo it.

These are pretty before and taste delicious after!

Crispy Romano Fritters with Fresh Tomato Slices

MAKES 4 FRITTERS

I like to serve these cheesy bites as an appetizer at Sunday brunch. You can dip them in marinara sauce—yum!

Vegetable or sesame oil, for the pan
2 large eggs
1 cup grated Romano cheese
6 tablespoons flour
Black pepper
2 tablespoons bread crumbs
8 thin tomato slices, for serving

EveryGirl

TIP: Use a small saucepan for this recipe so that you use less oil.

EveryGirl

TIP: The batter for the fritters is quite wet, so be sure to use well-floured hands to form the patties.

1. Add the oil to a small saucepan, about ½ inch up the sides, and warm the oil until hot but not smoking. Line a shallow bowl with paper towels.

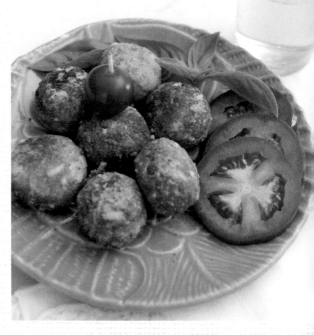

2. In a medium bowl, whisk the eggs until frothy. Fold in the cheese, 4 tablespoons of the flour, and a pinch of pepper. Form into 1-inch balls; roll the balls in the remaining 2 tablespoons flour and the bread crumbs. Gently flatten the balls into 3-inch patties. Drop the patties into the hot oil; cook for 3 minutes on each side, or until golden and crisp. Transfer to a paper towel–lined plate to absorb the excess oil. Serve the fritters with the sliced tomatoes.

Meatball Sliders

MAKES ABOUT 12 SLIDERS

I love making these for Super Bowl parties or any get-together where I don't want to make too many elaborate dishes. They are incredibly yummy and filling.

1 large egg, beaten

½ cup bread crumbs

1 pound ground beef

1 small onion, minced

2 teaspoons chopped fresh oregano

1 clove garlic, minced

1 teaspoon Worcestershire sauce

½ cup tomato sauce

Salt and black pepper

Olive oil, for frying

Small dinner rolls

Shredded Cheddar, ketchup, and mustard, for garnish

EveryGirl

TIP: Let the meatballs brown on one side before trying to turn them. Use tongs to gently roll them in the skillet. Don't squeeze them—the mixture is soft and the meatballs may crumble.

1. In a small bowl, whisk the egg. Place the bread crumbs in another bowl. In a large bowl, combine the beef, onion, oregano, garlic, Worcestershire sauce, tomato sauce, and salt and pepper to taste. Form into golf ball–sized balls. Coat the balls with the beaten egg, then the bread crumbs.

2. In a medium skillet over medium-high heat, pour the oil to reach about ½ inch up the sides of the pan. Cook the meatballs for about 10 minutes, turning until browned on all sides and cooked through. Sandwich the meatballs in rolls, garnishing with the Cheddar, ketchup, and mustard, as desired.

Feta Dip

SERVES 8   This recipe is diabetic-friendly and gluten-free!

Serve this creamy, spicy dip with crudités or pita crisps. Add as much or as little crushed red pepper as you like. Use it as a dip or a spread. Imagine this on your next chicken sandwich!

1 pound feta cheese, crumbled

⅓ cup olive oil

1 tablespoon crushed red pepper flakes, or to taste

Black pepper, to taste

Combine the cheese, oil, crushed red pepper, and black pepper in a food processor; puree until smooth.

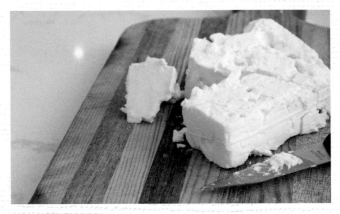

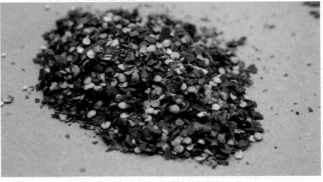

Feta-Avocado Dip

SERVES 12   This recipe is diabetic-friendly and gluten-free!

Two of my favorite ingredients whipped into one pretty green dip! Yum! I call this recipe the Greek guacamole!

1 pound feta cheese, crumbled

3 avocados, sliced

3 tablespoons olive oil

3 tablespoons fresh lemon juice (from 1 large lemon)

2 cloves garlic, minced

Salt and black pepper

Combine the cheese, avocados, oil, lemon juice, garlic, and salt and pepper to taste in a food processor; puree until smooth.

EveryGirl
TIP: A food processor makes quick work of this dip. If you don't have one, you can also mash by hand in a large bowl.

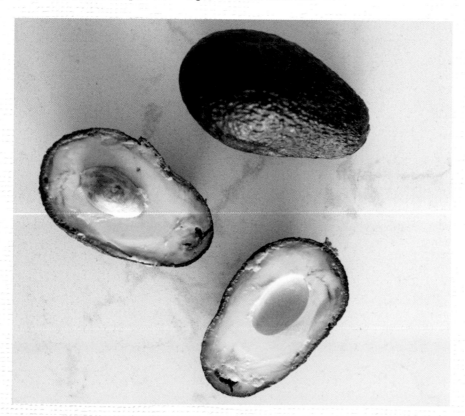

Yogurt-Cucumber Dip with Fresh Dill and Crudités

MAKES 1½ CUPS

This recipe is diabetic-friendly and gluten-free!

Serve this dip with whatever crudités you like best. If you don't have time to peel and chop veggies, pick up a bag of mini carrots.

EveryGirl

TIP: There's no need to peel the cucumber. The peel softens in the dip and adds pretty green flecks.

3 tablespoons extra-virgin olive oil

3 tablespoons fresh lemon juice (from 2 lemons)

½ teaspoon salt

1 small clove garlic, minced

2 tablespoons minced fresh dill

½ small cucumber, diced

1 cup plain nonfat Greek yogurt

Crudités, as desired

In a medium bowl, whisk the oil, lemon juice, salt, garlic, and dill. Fold in the cucumber and yogurt. Serve with crudités.

Olive-Feta Dip

MAKES 1½ CUPS   This recipe is diabetic-friendly and gluten-free!

This dip is super easy to make and endlessly versatile. Leftovers make a great sandwich spread or omelet filling.

    4 ounces (½ cup) pitted kalamata olives
    4 ounces (½ cup) crumbled feta cheese
    1 tablespoon chopped fresh oregano
    1 teaspoon granulated garlic
    ¼ cup extra-virgin olive oil

Combine the olives, cheese, oregano, granulated garlic, and olive oil in a food processor. Puree until creamy.

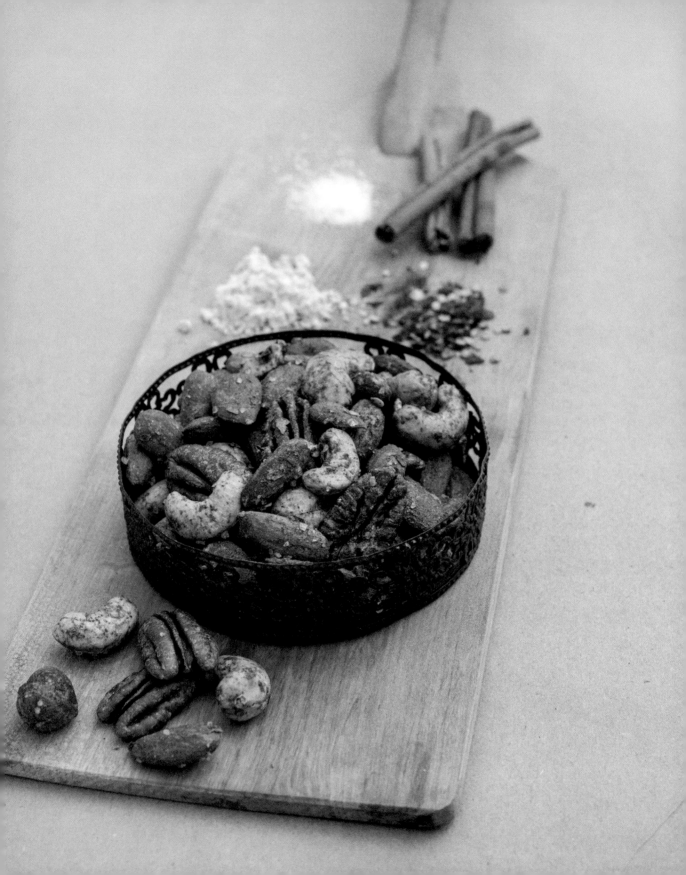

Spiced Mixed Nuts

MAKES 6 CUPS   This recipe is diabetic-friendly and gluten-free!

Okay, I know what you are thinking: "Who has time to make this when you can just buy a pre-made bag at the store?" Don't say that until you've tried it. These nuts are amazing! Make a huge batch and keep for nights you are entertaining, or times you want a little snack. Trust me, they are to die for!

- 2 egg whites
- 1½ teaspoons cinnamon
- 1½ teaspoons mustard powder
- 6 cups raw mixed nuts
- 1 to 1½ tablespoons kosher salt
- 1 tablespoon crushed red pepper

1. Preheat the oven to 250°F.

2. In a large bowl, beat the egg whites, add the cinnamon and mustard powder, then stir.

3. Add the nuts, salt, and red pepper. Stir to combine all the ingredients. Spread the mixture in a single layer on a large baking sheet.

4. Bake for 30 to 45 minutes, until lightly browned, stirring often. Let cool on the baking sheet.

EveryGirl **TIP:** Keep an eye on the nuts as they toast—they can burn quickly.

EveryGirl **TIP:** Kosher salt is a larger-grain variety, which works well in this dish. If all you have is table salt, use less—add it to taste.

EveryGirl **TIP:** Using raw nuts makes this a no-added-fat snack.

EveryGirl **TIP:** You can also use this recipe to make a pie crust (just smash the nuts).

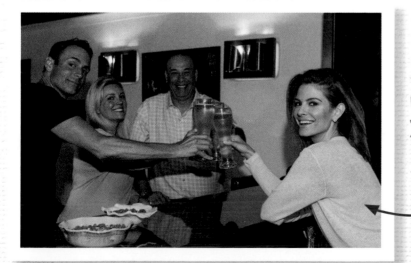

In our newly renovated home bar, courtesy of our friend, host of Spike TV's Bar Rescue, Jon Taffer. His wife, Nicole, Kev, and I toasting to good health!

Cucumber-Tomato-Feta Bites

MAKES 12 BITES   This recipe is diabetic-friendly and gluten-free!

Just because you are in a rush doesn't mean you can't have a little fun with your food. Who doesn't like to eat from a stick? This one is a total crowd-pleaser.

½ small cucumber, split and cut into medium slices

6 cherry tomatoes, cut in halves

3 ounces feta cheese, crumbled into bite size

½ red bell pepper, cut into ½-inch cubes

2 tablespoons extra-virgin olive oil

2 tablespoons lemon juice (if you prefer vinegar, use that)

Oregano

1. Using toothpicks, slide slices of the cucumber and tomatoes, the feta, and red pepper in alternating patterns onto the toothpicks.

2. Drizzle the veggies with the oil and lemon juice, and sprinkle with oregano.

EveryGirl

TIP: Don't cut the veggies too thick, otherwise your guests won't be able to grab them. Trust me, I've made that mistake!

EveryGirl

TIP: If you've got some fresh herbs, chop them up and sprinkle them over the kabobs before serving.

EveryGirl

TIP: Some people don't like the skin on the cucumber, but the skin is full of nutrients!

Compromise by running a fork down the length of the cucumber before slicing; this removes a little bit of the skin and looks pretty.

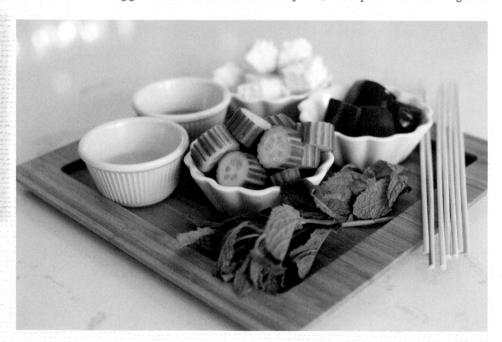

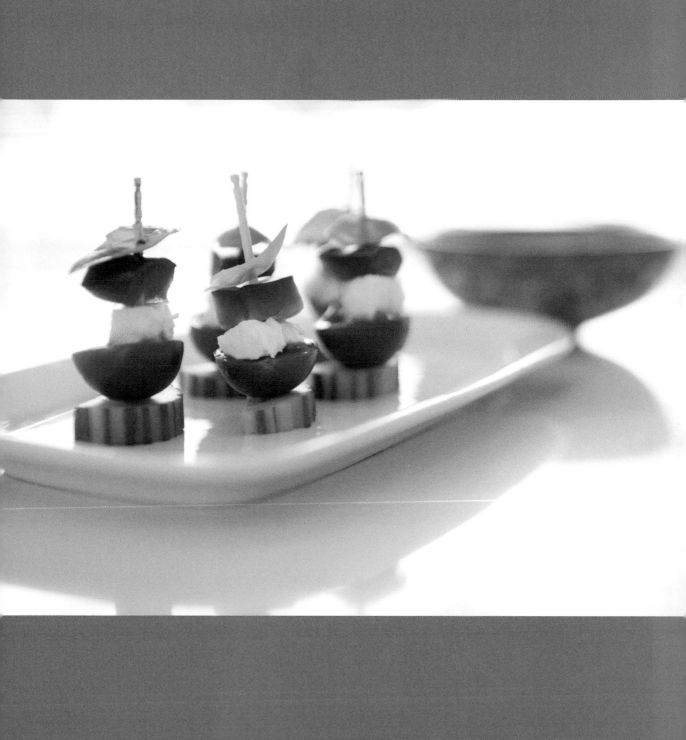

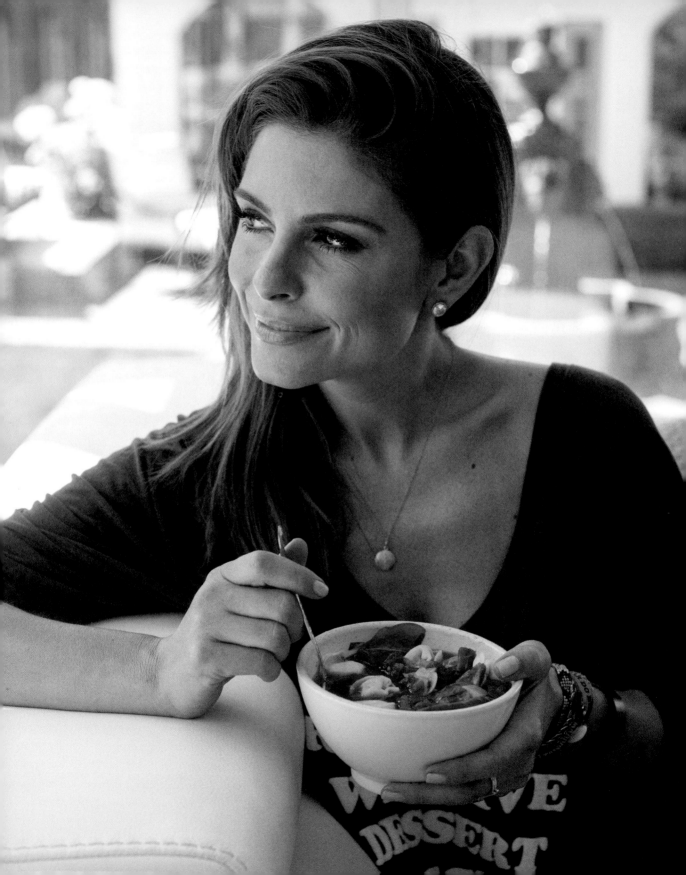

EveryGirl ENTERTAINS

Main Courses

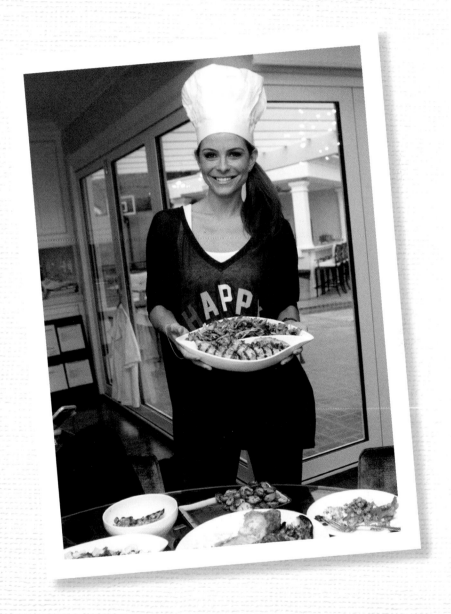

Orzo Picnic Salad

SERVES 6 TO 8   If you have just one serving, this recipe is diabetic-friendly! **Ⓓ**

Since this bright, crunchy salad offers an equal amount of pasta and veggies, you can satisfy your pasta cravings and fill up on healthy vegetables all in one meal! It's my go-to for a dinner party—everyone loves it and it looks super pretty!

8 ounces orzo

Dressing
⅓ cup extra-virgin olive oil
⅓ cup fresh lemon juice (from 3 lemons)
1 clove garlic, minced
Salt and black pepper

Salad
1 green bell pepper, diced
1 red bell pepper, diced
1 small cucumber, seeded and diced
½ cup chopped fresh parsley
½ cup chopped almonds
1 cup cherry tomatoes, halved
1 cup baby spinach, coarsely chopped

EveryGirl
TIP: If you can find it, use Greek orzo. Marinate the orzo and leave it overnight. And make extra so you can take some into the office the next day.

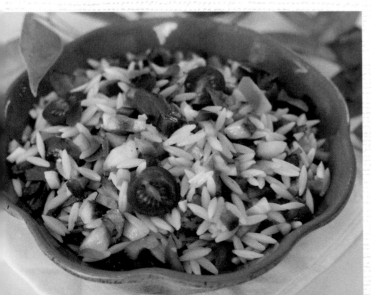

1. Cook the orzo according to the package directions. Drain and let cool.

2. In a large serving bowl, whisk the oil, lemon juice, garlic, and salt and pepper to taste until combined. Add the green and red bell peppers, cucumber, parsley, almonds, tomatoes, baby spinach, and cooled orzo; toss to combine.

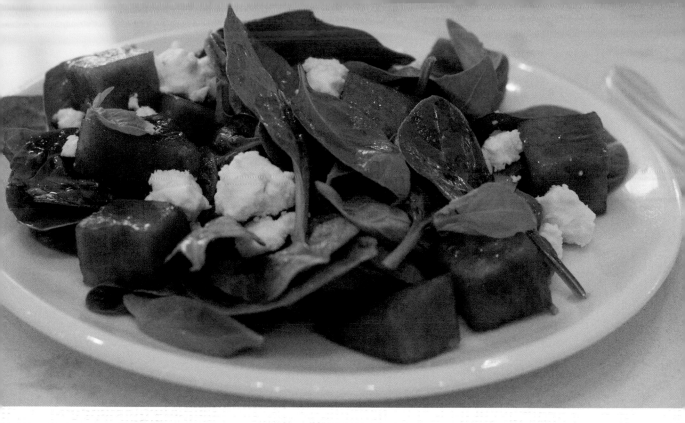

Summertime Watermelon-Feta Salad

SERVES 4

The vibrant colors in this salad make a stunning presentation!

- ¼ cup extra-virgin olive oil
- 2 tablespoons white wine vinegar or fresh lemon juice
- 3 cups cubed seedless watermelon
- ½ cup crumbled feta cheese
- 2 cups (about 2½ ounces) shredded spinach leaves
- ½ cup sliced fresh basil

EveryGirl
TIP: Make sure to cut the watermelon and spinach into small pieces; you want both flavors in every bite.

1. In a serving bowl, whisk the oil and vinegar until blended.

2. Add the watermelon, feta cheese, spinach, and basil; gently toss to combine.

Three-Cheese Eggplant Lasagna

SERVES 8 TO 10

Even though we are Greek, we still know how to make a cheesy, gooey, delicious lasagna.

3 cups part-skim ricotta cheese (24 ounces)
½ cup grated Parmesan cheese
1 large egg
Salt and black pepper
3 tablespoons olive oil
1 medium eggplant, thinly sliced (about 18 slices)
1 medium onion, chopped
4 cloves garlic, minced
3 tablespoons minced fresh basil or prepared basil pesto
1 can (28 ounces) tomato sauce
12 sheets oven-ready (no-boil) lasagna
2 cups shredded mozzarella cheese (about 1 pound)

EveryGirl
TIP: A glass baking dish is the best pan for lasagna. The acid in tomato sauce can react to metal. Furthermore, it's much easier to clean baked-on food from glass than metal.

1. Preheat the oven to 350°F.

2. In a medium bowl, whisk the ricotta, Parmesan, egg, and salt and pepper to taste.

3. Warm 1 tablespoon of the oil in a large skillet over medium heat. Add half of the eggplant slices in one layer and cook until lightly browned on both sides. Using tongs, transfer the slices to a platter. Add another 1 tablespoon oil and repeat the process with the remaining eggplant slices. Warm the remaining 1 tablespoon oil in the same skillet. Add the onion; cook for 5 minutes, stirring. Add the garlic; cook for 30 seconds, stirring. Remove from the heat; stir in the basil. Stir the skillet ingredients into the ricotta mixture.

4. In a 9 x 13-inch pan, layer the tomato sauce, noodles, eggplant, and ricotta mixture.

5. Repeat this layering two more times. Pour any leftover tomato sauce over the whole pan, especially along the sides. Cover the pan tightly with foil and bake for 30 minutes, or until the noodles are tender.

6. Remove the foil; sprinkle with the mozzarella and bake, uncovered, for 10 minutes, or until the mozzarella is melted.

Big Fat Greek Salad

SERVES 6   This recipe is diabetic-friendly and gluten-free!

In honor of my favorite Greek movie—My Big Fat Greek Wedding—here is my big fat Greek salad! It's always my go-to salad. I like to substitute scallions for the onion.

Dressing
½ cup extra-virgin olive oil
¼ cup fresh lemon juice (from 2 lemons)
1 small clove garlic, minced
1 teaspoon chopped fresh oregano

Salad
1 large head romaine lettuce, chopped
1 green bell pepper, sliced
1 red bell pepper, sliced
1 yellow bell pepper, sliced
½ cup capers
1 small cucumber, sliced
1 small red onion, sliced
½ cup pitted black olives
½ cup cubed feta cheese
2 medium tomatoes, diced

1. For the dressing, in a large serving bowl, whisk the oil, lemon juice, garlic, and oregano until combined.

2. For the salad, add the lettuce, green, red, and yellow bell peppers, capers, cucumber, onion, olives, feta, and tomatoes. Toss to coat.

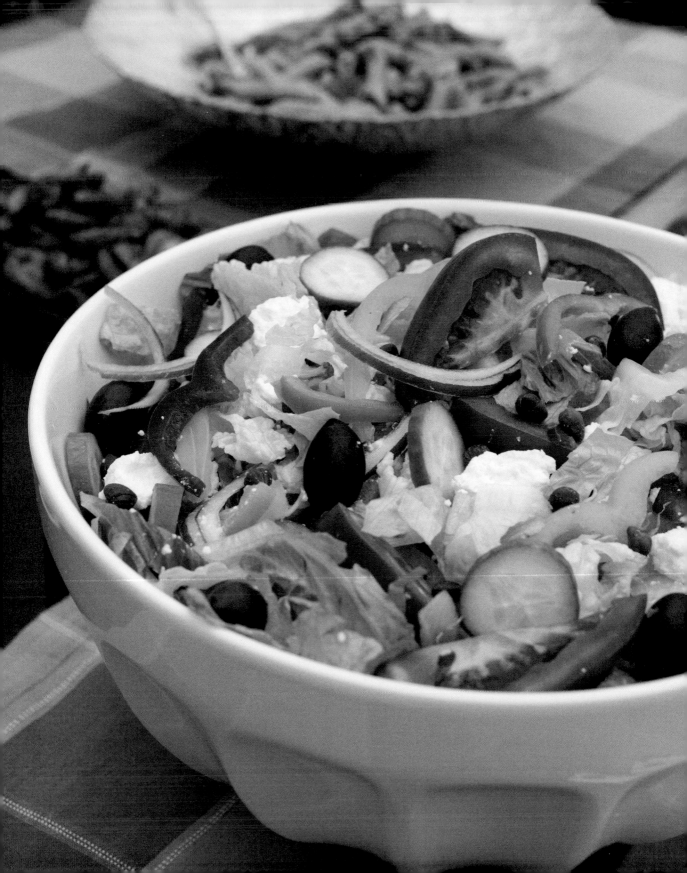

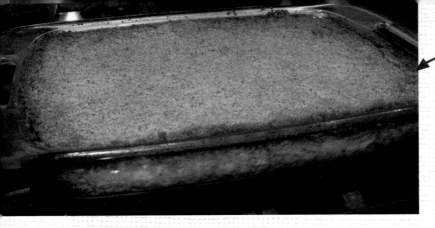

I made this for Thanksgiving this year!

Crabmeat Pie Lasagna

SERVES 4 TO 6

Your loved ones will get addicted to this and will start to get upset if you don't make it for them all the time. It is that good!

EveryGirl

TIP: You'll find cooked crabmeat in the refrigerated seafood aisle; try to avoid the canned crab.

EveryGirl

TIP: I always make extra bread crumbs and butter mixture because I don't like to run out and I also love the extra topping.

Crabmeat

1 pound cooked crabmeat

1½ cups milk, warmed

6 slices white bread, cubed

8 tablespoons (1 stick) unsalted butter, melted

Black pepper

Topping

1 cup unseasoned bread crumbs

4 tablespoons (½ stick) unsalted butter, melted

1. Preheat the oven to 350°F.

2. In a bowl, mix the crabmeat, milk, bread cubes, and butter and mush together with your hands.

3. Spread the crabmeat mixture in a pie pan. Season with pepper to taste.

4. For the topping, combine the bread crumbs and butter and sprinkle over the crabmeat mixture. Bake for 20 minutes, or until golden and hot.

Violeta's Fish Ceviche

SERVES 4 TO 6   This recipe is diabetic-friendly and gluten-free!

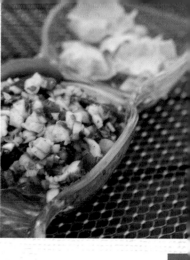

I learned this recipe from my longtime housekeeper and friend, Violeta.
I am so blessed to have her in my life; she is family.

8 ounces tilapia

½ cup lemon juice (fresh or bottled)

4 tomatoes

½ white onion

2 Persian cucumbers

½ bunch cilantro

1 to 2 fresh jalapeño peppers (depends on how spicy you want the dish)

1½ teaspoons salt

½ teaspoon black pepper

Dash of oregano

1. Thinly slice the fish (don't chop) and place it in a deep dish. Cover with the lemon juice. Leave in the fridge for 1 hour.

2. Chop up the tomatoes, onion, cucumbers, cilantro, and jalapeños.

3. Drain the lemon juice from the fish and cut the fish into small pieces. In a bowl, combine the vegetables and fish. Season with the salt, pepper, and oregano.

EveryGirl

TIP: For a pool party or afternoon gathering, I like to make this because it's light and delicious. Serve with tortilla chips or on top of small lettuce wraps.

EveryGirl

TIP: Fresh fish is always the best, but you can also find tilapia in the frozen food aisle.

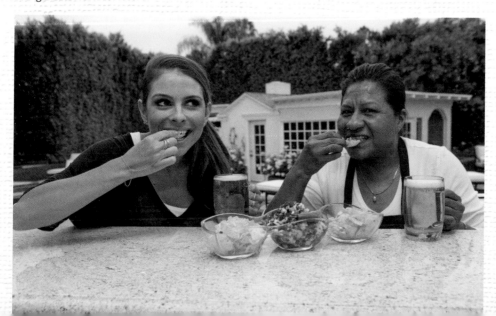

Chive-Roasted Fingerling Potatoes

SERVES 3 TO 4

These are to-die-for delicious, so be careful—you could easily go crazy and eat the entire dish yourself!

1 pound fingerling potatoes, halved
3 tablespoons olive oil
2 tablespoons chopped fresh chives
Salt and black pepper

1. Preheat the oven to 425°F. Place a baking sheet in the oven to heat.

2. In a large bowl, toss the potatoes, oil, chives, and salt and pepper to taste until coated.

3. Remove the sheet from the oven; spread the potatoes onto the sheet. Return the sheet to the oven and roast the potatoes for 20 minutes, or until crispy on the outside and tender inside. Stir the potatoes or shake the pan several times during roasting to brown all sides.

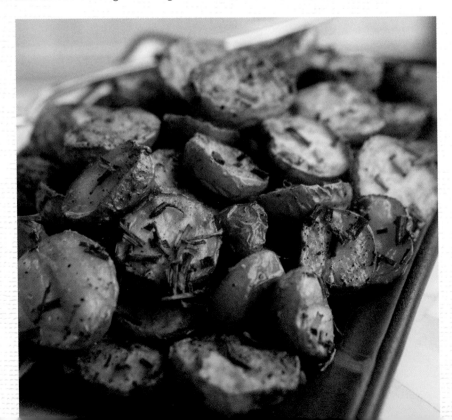

Another cooking legend is the great Giada De Laurentiis. Giada is a dear friend and certified culinary genius. Giada has been to my house for Thanksgiving! I can't tell you the stress I felt knowing someone of her level was going to see me in action in the kitchen. But Giada, being Giada, was incredibly supportive, as she has been throughout our friendship—and grateful. She appreciated, for once, NOT having the pressure to cook for everyone on a holiday. She also educated my Italian American boyfriend, Kev, on the difference between Neapolitan Italian food here in America and Italian food in Italy.

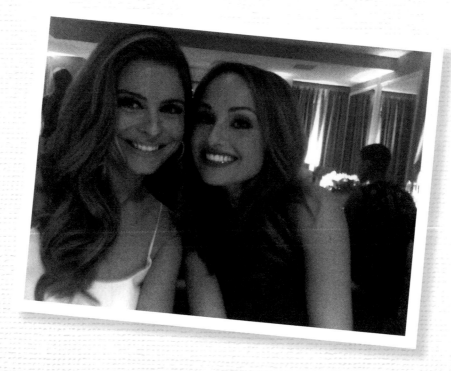

I love getting to spend time with Giada. She has been such a great friend. Here we are at a dinner in Los Angeles.

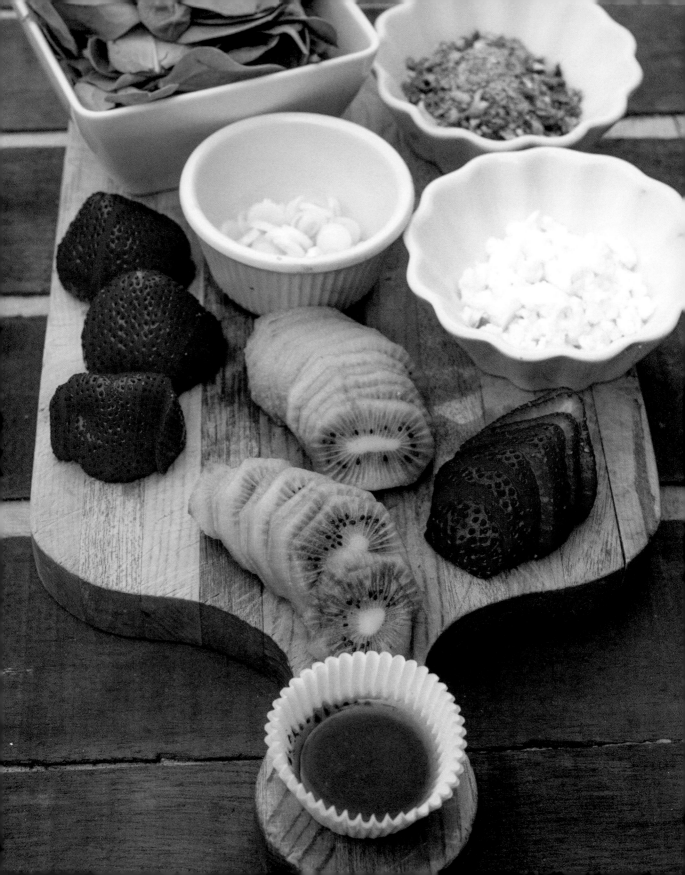

Spinach-Kiwi Salad with Salted Pistachios

SERVES 2   This recipe is diabetic-friendly and gluten-free!

Feel free to use your dressing of choice for this recipe, but trust me that this simple oil-and-vinegar one is all these vibrant and tasty ingredients need! You can prep all the components of this salad in advance, but wait to toss everything together until just before serving.

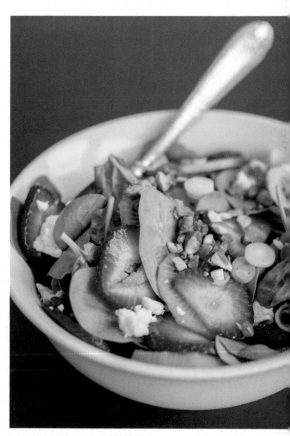

Dressing
1 tablespoon extra-virgin olive oil
2 teaspoons balsamic vinegar

Salad
4 cups baby spinach (2½ ounces)
2 kiwis, peeled and sliced
4 strawberries, sliced
1 scallion (white and light green parts only), thinly
    sliced
¼ cup crumbled feta or goat cheese
¼ cup chopped salted pistachios
Salt and black pepper

1. In a medium serving bowl, whisk the oil and vinegar.

2. Add the spinach, kiwis, strawberries, scallion, feta, and pistachios; toss to coat.

3. Season with salt and pepper to taste.

Late Summer Quinoa Salad with Black Beans, Charred Corn, and Honey-Lime Vinaigrette

SERVES 4 TO 6

You can make this salad in advance, but wait to fold in the avocado and cilantro until just before serving.

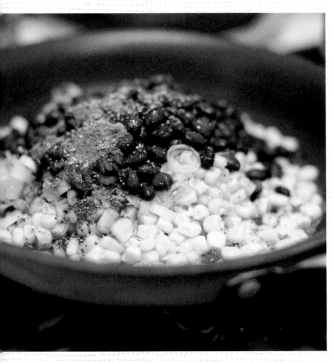

1 cup quinoa

3 ears corn, kernels cut off cob

3 scallions (white and light green parts only), thinly sliced

1 cup drained canned black beans

2 teaspoons ground cumin

½ mango, chopped

3 tablespoons extra-virgin olive oil

2 tablespoons fresh lime juice (from 1 lime)

2 teaspoons honey or agave

Salt

Cayenne pepper

1 avocado, diced

3 medium tomatoes, seeded and diced (about 1½ cups)

½ cup chopped fresh cilantro

EveryGirl
TIP: Use a serrated knife (knife with a jagged edge) to cut the kernels from the corn.

1. Cook the quinoa according to the package directions. Transfer to a large serving bowl.

2. Warm a large skillet over medium heat. Add the corn kernels; cook for 4 minutes, or until lightly charred, stirring. Stir in the scallions, beans, cumin, and mango, stirring to warm through. Add to the quinoa. Add the oil, lime juice, honey, and salt and cayenne pepper to taste; toss to coat. Fold in the avocado, tomatoes, and cilantro.

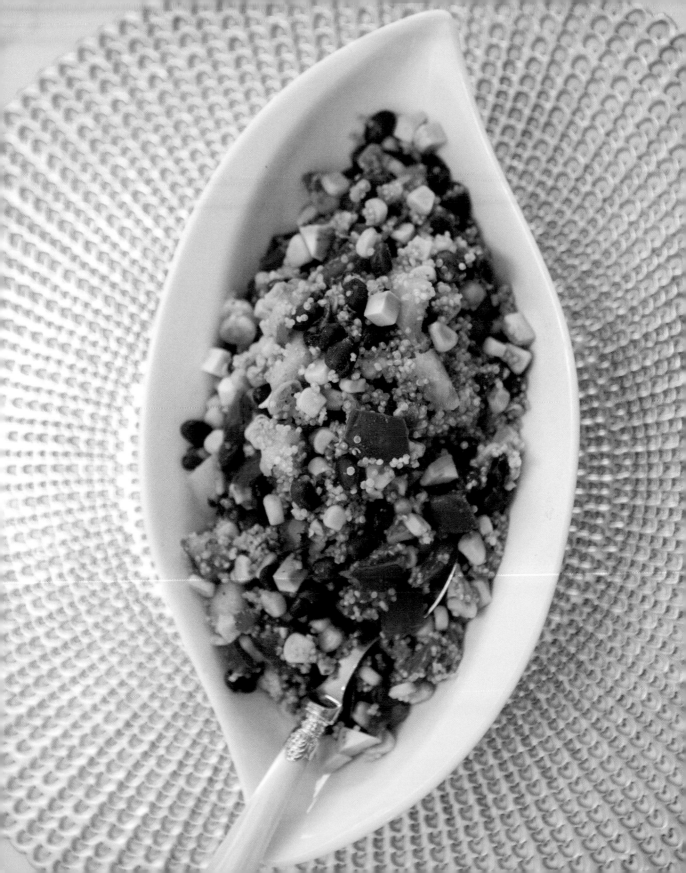

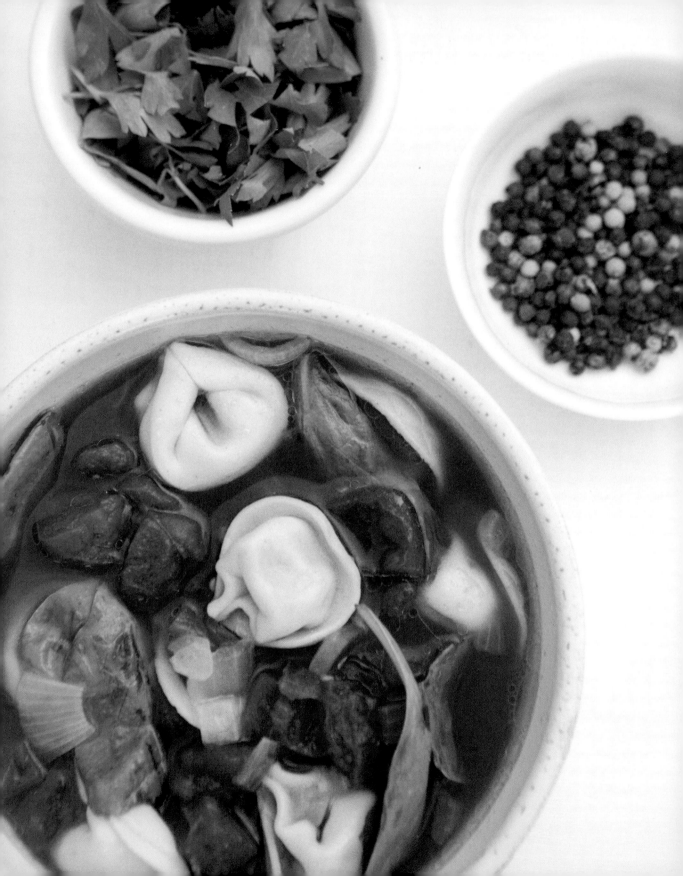

Fresh Tomato and Spinach Soup with Tortellini

SERVES 4

I die for this soup. It's another staple for my dinner parties because it's fresh and looks beautiful on the table. You will never disappoint with this recipe! It's best made in the summer, when tomatoes are farm fresh.

2 tablespoons olive oil

1 large shallot or 1 small onion, chopped

3 cloves garlic, minced

4 cups (32 ounces) vegetable or chicken broth

6 ounces fresh cheese tortellini

1¾ pounds fresh tomatoes (about 4 medium tomatoes), chopped

1 box (5 ounces) baby or regular spinach

1. Warm the oil in a large saucepan or Dutch oven over medium heat.

2. Add the shallot; cook for 5 minutes, until softened, stirring.

3. Add the garlic; cook for 30 seconds, stirring.

4. Add the broth and tortellini; cook for 5 minutes.

5. Stir in the tomatoes and spinach; cook until the spinach is wilted and the soup is warmed through.

EveryGirl TIP: Feel free to substitute any flavor tortellini or ravioli in the soup.

EveryGirl TIP: Pre-washed baby spinach leaves are the easiest to use, but are more expensive than a regular bunch of spinach. You can always substitute regular spinach, but remember to trim off the stems and wash and chop the leaves before adding to a recipe.

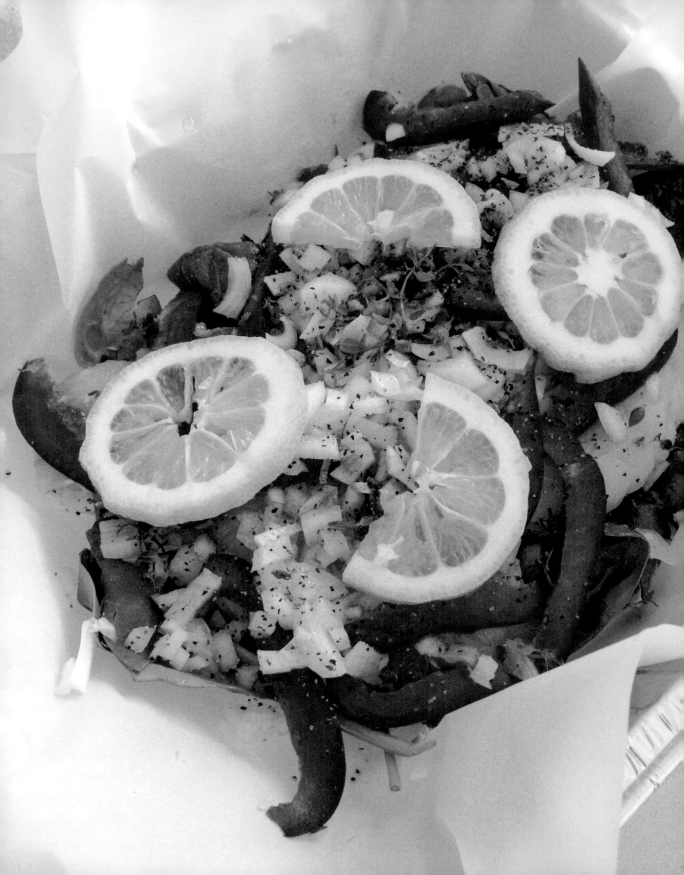

My Cousin Tashi's Halibut

SERVES 4   This recipe is diabetic-friendly and gluten-free!

My cousin Tashi is a sous chef in Boston at the Omni Parker House Hotel. He got the chef bug from my grandfather and his parents as well, who were also great cooks. We worked together at his dad's restaurant, Pete's Sunrise Restaurant, in Everett, Massachusetts. He cooked; I waitressed. He's really talented and I wanted to share this delicious and super-simple, yet super-impressive, recipe with all of you.

1 cup fresh spinach

6 to 8 ounces halibut

½ small red bell pepper, sliced

½ small onion, sliced

Sprig of fresh thyme

1 lemon, sliced (save some for garnish)

Sea salt and black pepper

Olive oil

EveryGirl
TIP: You can add different types of vegetables or fish, to make this dish your own. It's a quick and healthy meal that will impress everyone!

1. Preheat the oven to 450°F. Cut a large piece of parchment paper. Place the spinach down the middle of the paper first, then add the halibut. Place the red pepper, onion, thyme sprig, and lemon slices on top of the fish. Sprinkle with salt and pepper and a drizzle of olive oil.

2. Fold the parchment paper over and crimp the two sides together. This will also work just fine with aluminum foil. Place the fish package in a baking pan and bake for 20 to 25 minutes. Cut open the paper right before serving on a plate. Garnish with the reserved lemon slices.

Love my cousin Tashi!

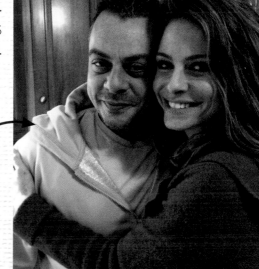

Eggplant-Potato Casserole

Serve this rustic dish directly out of the cast-iron skillet. Just remember to set it on a trivet or hot pad to protect your table.

¼ cup olive oil

2 medium onions, thinly sliced

1 cup tomato sauce

½ cup chopped fresh basil (about 9 leaves)

3 cloves garlic, minced

Salt and black pepper

2 medium red or Yukon Gold potatoes, *very thinly* sliced

1 medium eggplant, thinly sliced

½ cup bread crumbs (if you want a lower-calorie dish, omit the bread crumbs)

EveryGirl

TIP: No need to peel the eggplant, but it's best to use a serrated knife for slicing.

1. Preheat the oven to 350°F.

2. Warm 2 tablespoons of the oil in a medium saucepan over medium-low heat. Add the onions; cook for 10 minutes, stirring often. Add the tomato sauce, basil, garlic, and salt and pepper to taste, then add ½ cup water. Cook for 5 minutes, stirring.

3. Drizzle 1 tablespoon of the oil in the bottom of a 10-inch cast-iron or heavy ovenproof skillet. Layer the potatoes, eggplant, and prepared sauce, then repeat. Pour any remaining sauce over the top of the vegetables. Tightly cover the pan with foil; bake for 20 minutes.

4. Toss the bread crumbs with the remaining 1 tablespoon oil. Sprinkle the casserole with the bread crumbs. Bake, uncovered, for 15 minutes, or until the vegetables are tender.

Fettuccine Alfredo

SERVES 4

This creamy sauce couldn't be quicker—it cooks in less time than it takes to cook the pasta. I've added peas for a splash of green, but you could add a different vegetable or your choice of cooked meat or fish.

12 ounces fettuccine (regular, whole-wheat, or rice)
8 tablespoons (1 stick) unsalted butter
2 large cloves garlic, peeled and smashed
1 cup half-and-half
1 cup frozen peas
2 cups grated Parmesan cheese
Black pepper

EveryGirl
TIP: To make a spicy Alfredo sauce, just stir in a teaspoon of crushed red pepper.

1. Cook the pasta according to the package directions. Drain, reserving ¼ cup of the cooking water.

2. Melt the butter in a medium saucepan over medium-low heat. Add the garlic, half-and-half, peas, and cheese. Cook until the cheese is melted, stirring often.

3. In a large bowl, toss the pasta with the sauce, adding the reserved cooking water as needed for the desired consistency. Season with pepper to taste.

Warm Butternut Squash and Roasted Cauliflower

SERVES 4

This recipe is diabetic-friendly and gluten-free!

This is a great side dish for a dinner party or even for a solo dinner party! It's delicious and easy to pack in a small Tupperware to take to work or to have as leftovers the next day.

Cauliflower

1 small (¼ pound) butternut squash, peeled and cut into ¾-inch chunks

3 tablespoons olive oil

Salt and black pepper

½ large head cauliflower, cut into florets

Dressing

3 tablespoons extra-virgin olive oil

2 tablespoons fresh lemon juice (from 1 lemon)

1 teaspoon white wine vinegar

¼ to ½ teaspoon paprika

Salt and black pepper

2 scallions (white and light green parts only), sliced

2 tablespoons finely chopped fresh mint leaves

2 tablespoons, finely chopped fresh parsley or cilantro

¼ cup salted pumpkin seeds (*pepitos*)

1. Preheat the oven to 375°F.

2. Spread out the cubed squash in a single layer on a baking sheet; drizzle with 2 tablespoons of the oil, and salt and pepper to taste. Roast for 30 to 35 minutes, until tender.

3. Spread out the cauliflower on a second baking sheet in a single layer and drizzle with the remaining 1 tablespoon of oil; season with salt and pepper to taste. Roast for 20 minutes, or until tender-crisp, stirring occasionally.

4. For the dressing, in a large bowl, whisk together the 3 tablespoons of oil, the lemon juice, vinegar, paprika, and salt and pepper to taste.

5. To serve, fold the squash, cauliflower, scallions, mint, and parsley into the dressing. Season with salt and pepper to taste. Garnish with the pumpkin seeds.

EveryGirl
TIP: Save time by using pre-cut squash cubes. Just make sure you buy ones that look fresh.

Grilled Balsamic Chicken with Party Potato Salad

SERVES 4

This is a great dish for any occasion. It takes "everyday chicken" to another level.

Marinade
¼ cup balsamic vinegar

2 tablespoons Dijon mustard

2 cloves garlic, minced

2 tablespoons fresh lime juice (from 1 lime)

Salt and black pepper

4 boneless, skinless chicken breast halves

Potato Salad
1 pound red potatoes, unpeeled and diced

5 tablespoons extra-virgin olive oil

3 tablespoons red wine vinegar

1 small red onion, diced

1 small green bell pepper, diced

1 small yellow bell pepper, diced

1 cup baby spinach, sliced

¼ cup crumbled feta cheese

½ cup chopped fresh parsley

Salt and black pepper

EveryGirl

TIP: You can make the potato salad a day in advance. Store, tightly covered, in the refrigerator. You can also get the chicken marinating a day in advance. Let it sit at room temperature for at least 20 minutes before grilling.

1. In a large glass bowl, whisk the balsamic vinegar, mustard, garlic, lime juice, and salt and pepper to taste. Reserve ¼ cup and set aside. Add the chicken to the marinade in the bowl; turn to coat. Refrigerate for at least 20 minutes and up to 12 hours.

2. Preheat the grill to medium-high heat. Grill the chicken, brushing on the reserved marinade in the first 5 minutes of cooking. Transfer to a cutting board to rest.

3. Meanwhile, in a medium saucepan, cook the potatoes in salted water to cover for 10 minutes, or until tender. Drain; transfer to a large bowl. Fold in the oil and vinegar. Fold in the onion, bell peppers, spinach, feta, and parsley, and season with salt and pepper to taste.

4. Serve the chicken with the potato salad warm or at room temperature.

Sloppy BBQ Buns with Cabbage Coleslaw

SERVES 4   Use a whole-wheat bun and this recipe is diabetic-friendly! **D**

When you want something hearty and flavorful, this is your dish! I especially love this when it's cold outside! Keep a wet napkin close—things tend to get messy. In the best possible way.

Sandwiches
1 tablespoon olive oil
1 medium onion, minced
1 pound ground beef
2 tablespoons Worcestershire sauce
2 tablespoons red-wine vinegar
1 tablespoon brown sugar
½ cup ketchup
¼ cup water
Salt
Whole-wheat or gluten-free buns or bread

Coleslaw
¼ cup olive oil
2 tablespoons rice-wine, white-wine, or apple-cider vinegar
3 cloves garlic, minced
Salt and black pepper
½ green cabbage, shredded
½ red cabbage, shredded

EveryGirl
TIP: If you like your BBQ sauce spicy, add a teaspoon of cayenne pepper.

EveryGirl
TIP: Save time by using a 16-ounce bag of fresh cabbage mix in place of the green and red cabbages.

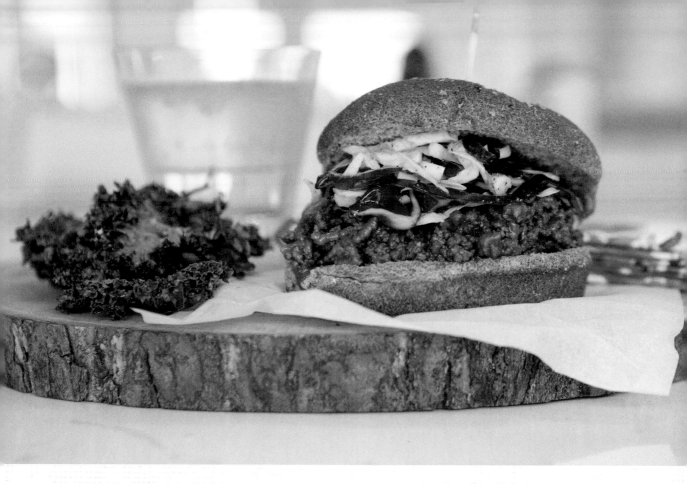

1. For the sandwiches, warm the oil in a large cast-iron or heavy skillet over medium heat. Add the onion; cook for 5 minutes, stirring. Increase the heat to medium-high; add the beef and cook for 6 minutes, until browned, stirring. Add the Worcestershire, vinegar, brown sugar, ketchup, and water; bring to a simmer. Reduce the heat and simmer for 8 minutes, stirring occasionally and adding water if needed. Season to taste with salt. Spoon the filling into the buns.

2. For the coleslaw, in a large bowl, whisk the oil, vinegar, garlic, and salt and pepper to taste. Add the shredded cabbage; toss to coat.

Eggplant Boats Stuffed with Lamb and Rice

SERVES 6

This recipe is diabetic-friendly and gluten-free!

My mom has always made these with lamb, but you can switch it up. I love serving these on a night when Keven and I have another couple over for dinner. It's impressive and filling.

3 medium eggplants, halved lengthwise

1 tablespoon olive oil, plus extra for brushing

Salt and black pepper

1 medium onion, diced

8 ounces ground lamb

1 cup tomato sauce

½ cup cooked rice

½ cup minced fresh parsley or basil

3 cloves garlic, minced

½ teaspoon ground cumin

½ teaspoon ground cinnamon

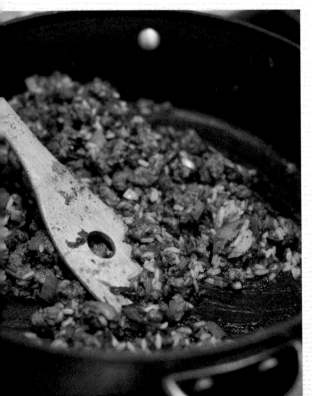

1. Preheat the oven to 400°F. Brush the flesh side of the eggplants with oil. Season with salt and pepper to taste. Place oiled-side down in a large roasting pan. Roast for 25 minutes, or until softened. Let cool. Reduce the oven temperature to 350°F.

2. Meanwhile, warm the 1 tablespoon of oil in a large skillet over medium-low heat. Cook the onion for 5 minutes, or until softened, stirring. Stir in the lamb, tomato sauce, cooked rice, parsley, garlic, cumin, cinnamon, and salt and pepper to taste. Cook for 5 minutes, stirring to break up the meat.

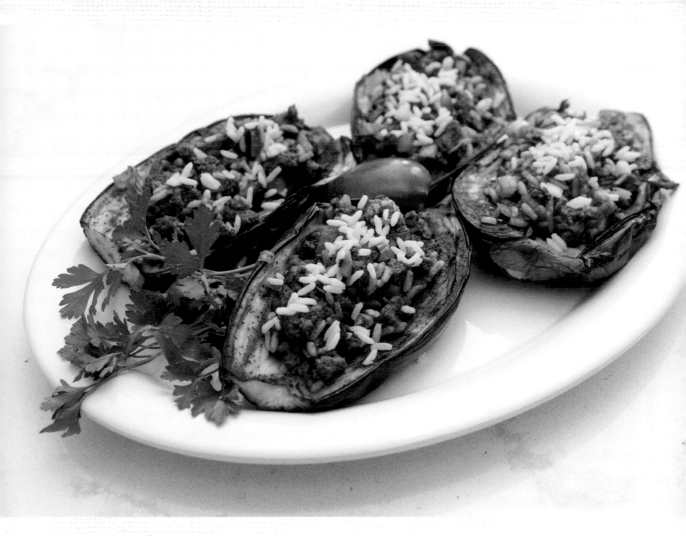

3. Carefully scoop out about half of the insides of the roasted eggplants; dice the insides and add to the skillet and stir. Spoon the mixture into the hollowed-out eggplants. Return the eggplant boats to the same roasting pan, filled side up. Cover the pan tightly with foil and roast for 50 minutes to 1 hour, until the eggplants are soft and the filling is hot.

EveryGirl
TIP: If you do not like lamb, you can use ground beef or turkey.

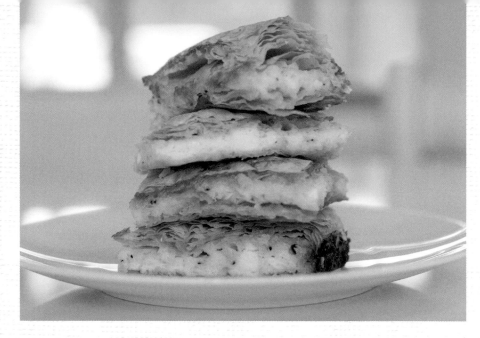

EveryGirl

TIP: Although white pepper looks better against the white of the cheese, black pepper is a perfectly fine substitute.

EveryGirl

TIP: You can put the pie together 1 day ahead; just cover it tightly and refrigerate. Bring to room temperature before baking.

If you don't want to deal with filo, you can use puff pastry sheets instead. Just spoon the mixture into the shells after the shells have risen a bit in the oven.

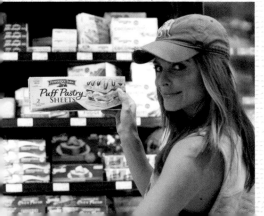

Tiropita (Golden Cheese Pie)

SERVES 12 TO 16

This is a traditional Greek dish that everyone in my family loves. It's very "splurgy," but so worth it!

5 large eggs

2 cups (about 8 ounces) crumbled feta cheese

1 cup grated Romano or Parmesan cheese

1 cup part-skim ricotta cheese

White pepper

¼ teaspoon ground nutmeg

½ pound filo dough (20 sheets)

1 cup (2 sticks) unsalted butter, melted

1. Preheat the oven to 350°F.

2. In a large bowl, whisk the eggs. Stir in the feta cheese, Romano cheese, and ricotta, season with the pepper, and add the nutmeg until blended.

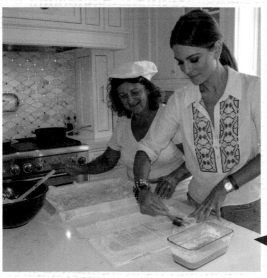

3. Lay 1 filo sheet in the bottom of a 9 x 13-inch pan, letting the ends of the sheet hang over the edges of the pan. Brush well with the butter. Top with 9 more sheets of filo, buttering between each sheet.

EveryGirl
TIP: Dampen a towel and place over the filo while you butter the sheets in the pan. If the filo is too dry, it will never be easy to work sheet by sheet. Filo must be room temperature when you remove the plastic packaging, and each sheet must be buttered.

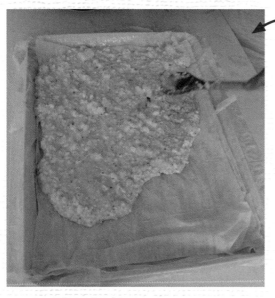

4. Spoon the cheese filling over the filo and fold the overhanging edges over the filling. Place 10 more sheets of filo over the filling, brushing with butter between each sheet. Butter the top sheet.

EveryGirl
TIP: Always buy 2 pounds of filo dough so if it's dry you have extra sheets. Always check the dates to ensure freshness. You can still use dry filo but it is harder to work with. Try to use unbroken sheets for the top layers, so it looks pretty.

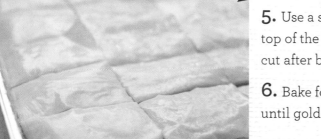

5. Use a sharp knife to score the top of the pie to make it easier to cut after baking.

6. Bake for about 40 minutes, or until golden brown.

Spanakopita (Greek Spinach Pie)

SERVES 12 TO 16

Serve this dish any time, at any temperature, for any occasion. Breakfast, brunch, lunch, appetizer, or dinner—it's always a hit!

2 tablespoons olive oil

2 pounds fresh spinach (about 3 big bunches), trimmed and chopped

4 scallions (white and light green parts only), sliced

½ head fennel, trimmed and chopped

¼ cup chopped fresh mint or dill

¼ cup chopped fresh parsley

Salt and black pepper

4 large eggs

1 cup crumbled feta cheese

½ cup part-skim ricotta cheese

1 pound filo dough (20 sheets), thawed to room temperature

1 cup (2 sticks) unsalted butter, melted

EveryGirl

TIP: For ease in preparation, use fresh spinach. Frozen spinach contains too much water. You can add the leaves to the skillet while still wet from washing. If you're in a real hurry, you can find Maria's Greek Delights at specialty and natural food retailers. If your local stores don't carry them yet, ask the managers to start stocking them!

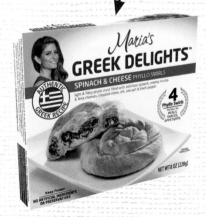

1. Preheat the oven to 350°F.

2. Warm the oil in a large skillet over medium-low heat. Add the spinach, scallions, and fennel; cook for 5 minutes, stirring. Stir in the mint, parsley, and salt and pepper to taste.

3. In a large bowl, whisk the eggs, feta, and ricotta until blended. Fold in the spinach mixture.

4. Lay 1 filo sheet in the bottom of a 9 x 13-inch pan, letting the ends of the sheet hang over the edges of the pan. Brush well with the butter. Top with 9 more filo sheets, buttering between each sheet.

5. Spoon the spinach filling over the filo and fold the overhanging edges over the filling. Place 10 more sheets of filo over the filling, brushing with the butter between each sheet.

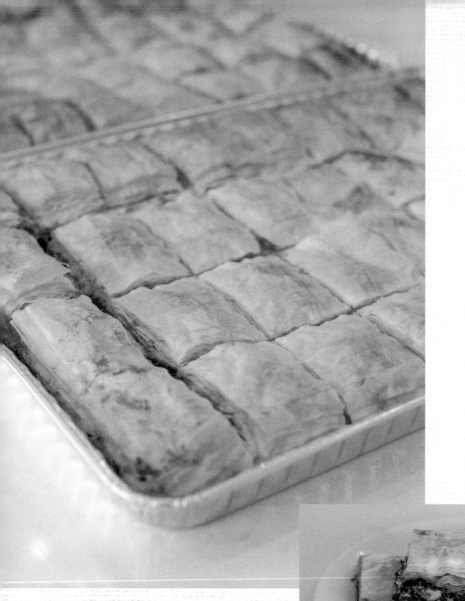

EveryGirl

TIP: For mini appetizers, drop a spoonful of the filling into prepared puff pastry shells and bake according to the package directions.

EveryGirl

TIP: Always buy 2 pounds of filo so if it's dry, you have extra sheets. Always check the dates to ensure freshness. You can still use dry filo but it is harder to work with. Try to use unbroken sheets for the top layers, so it looks pretty.

6. Butter the top sheet. Use a sharp knife to score the top of the pie to make it easier to cut after baking.

7. Bake for 40 minutes, or until golden brown.

Potluck Pesto, Potato, and Green Bean Salad

SERVES 4

Talk about easy and fast! This one has it all. And there's no need to peel the potatoes—in fact, the red skins look lovely against the green beans.

1½ pounds small red potatoes, quartered

8 ounces green beans, trimmed and halved

3 tablespoons white wine vinegar

3 scallions (white and light green parts only), thinly sliced

½ cup prepared or homemade basil pesto

Salt and black pepper

¼ cup chopped walnuts

In a medium saucepan, cook the potatoes in salted water for 12 to 15 minutes, until tender but still firm. Add the beans in the last 2 minutes of cooking. Drain. In a large bowl, toss the warm vegetables with the vinegar. Fold in the scallions and pesto. Season with salt and pepper to taste. Garnish with the nuts.

EveryGirl

TIP: The salad can be served warm, cool, or at room temperature. If you are making it in advance, wait to add the walnuts until just before serving.

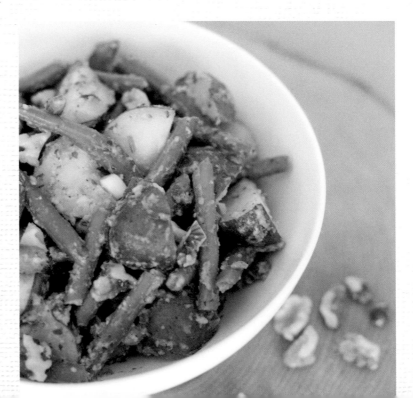

EveryGirl CELEBRITY COOKING MOMENT

One of my more fun moments at work was when I got to interview cooking icon Wolfgang Puck, and even work under him on a segment for *Access Hollywood*. He taught me several cool culinary tips, including the key to making a delicious burger. In addition to forming the burger patty itself, he recommended putting a good amount of salt and pepper on the patty before grilling. It vastly enhances the flavor in the easiest of ways.

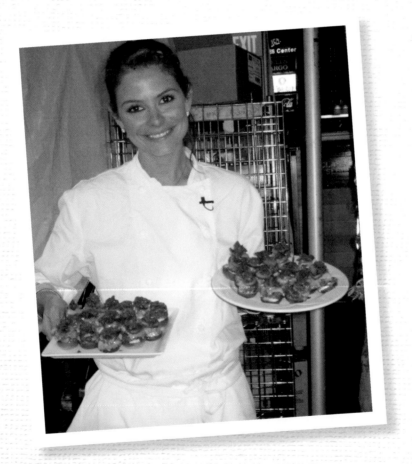

These are the mini burgers Wolfgang is famous for making after all the big Hollywood award shows!

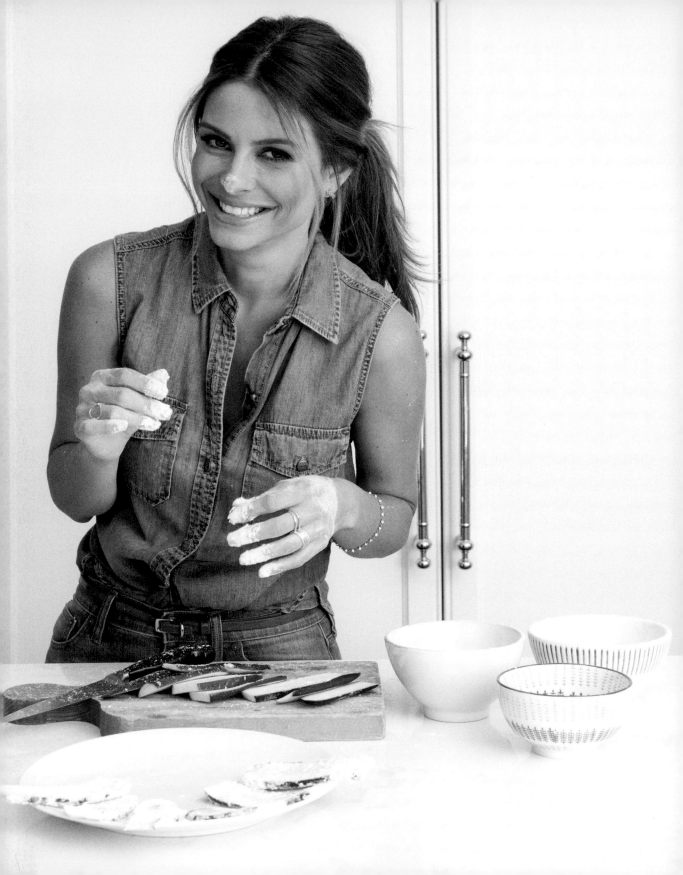

Everygirl

PATTIES GALORE

Mom and I love making patties. We make all different kinds, so I decided rather than choosing just one, I'd include all my favorite ones in this chapter. Patties are great finger foods/appetizers and most go great with Tzatziki (see page 202).

In the summer when I have extra veggies like zucchini, I shred them and freeze them, making these recipes even easier to prepare.

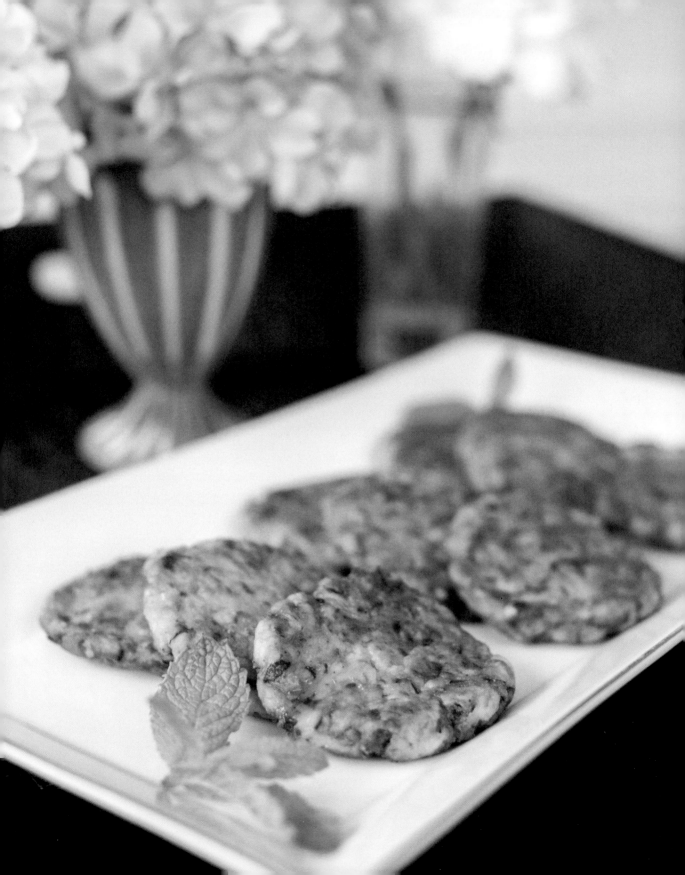

Cauliflower Patties

MAKES 25-30 PIECES   This recipe is diabetic-friendly! **Ⓓ**

1 head cauliflower, chopped and boiled until tender
1 large onion, minced
1 large egg
½ cup bread crumbs
½ cup minced fresh parsley
3 cloves garlic, minced
Salt and black pepper
1 cup all-purpose flour
Olive oil, for frying

1. In a large bowl drain the boiled cauliflower, then mash the cauliflower. Fold in the onion, egg, bread crumbs, parsley, garlic, and salt and pepper.

2. Scoop up a heaping tablespoon of the mixture. Form into a ball, then flatten with your palms.

3. Flour the patties on both sides.

4. Warm oil to about a half inch up the sides of a large skillet over medium-high heat. Cook the patties until golden brown on each side.

5. Transfer to a paper towel–lined plate until ready to serve.

EveryGirl
TIP: Transfer the hot patties to a paper towel–lined plate to soak up some of the cooking oil.

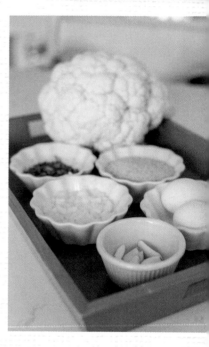

EveryGirl
TIP: Make the patties look more appealing and fancy by serving them on a pie plate.

Sweet Potato Patties

MAKES ABOUT 30 PATTIES

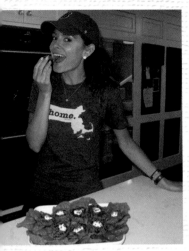

3 medium sweet potatoes, unpeeled

1½ tablespoons unsalted butter, at room temperature

1½ cups bread crumbs

½ medium onion, chopped

½ cup finely chopped almonds

1 teaspoon cinnamon

½ teaspoon crushed red pepper flakes

Salt

1 cup all-purpose flour

Olive oil, for frying

EveryGirl

TIP: With all patties, if consistency is too mushy to form a patty, add more bread crumbs.

EveryGirl

TIP: Always bake sweet potatoes in their skins; this will keep them moist and flavorful.

1. Preheat the oven to 350°F.

2. Bake the sweet potatoes for 40 minutes, or until soft. Remove from the oven and let cool slightly. Halve lengthwise and scoop out the flesh.

3. In a large bowl, mash the sweet potatoes. Fold in the butter, bread crumbs, onion, almonds, cinnamon, crushed red pepper, and salt to taste.

4. Using your hands, form small balls. Flatten into patties with your palms.

5. Flour the patties on both sides.

6. Warm oil to about a half inch up the sides of a large skillet over medium-high heat. Cook the patties until golden brown on each side.

7. Transfer to a paper towel–lined plate until ready to serve.

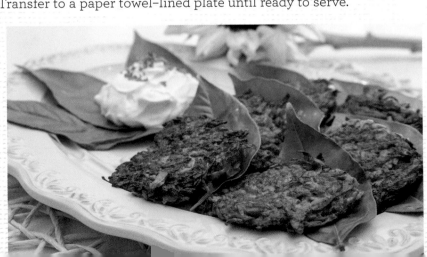

Spicy Zucchini Patties

MAKES ABOUT 30 PATTIES

This recipe is diabetic-friendly! **D**

4 zucchini, shredded

1 tablespoon salt

2 large eggs

1 cup bread crumbs

½ cup chopped fresh mint

1 tablespoon crushed red pepper flakes

Salt and black pepper

1 cup all-purpose flour

Olive oil, for frying

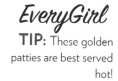

EveryGirl

TIP: These golden patties are best served hot!

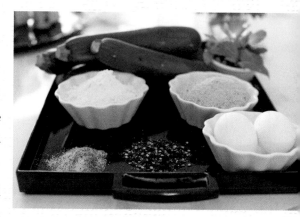

1. In a large bowl, toss the zucchini with the salt. Use your hands to squeeze as much water from the zucchini as possible. Drain the water from the bowl.

2. Fold in the eggs, bread crumbs, mint, crushed red pepper, and salt and pepper to taste. Using your hands, squish the mixture to a mushlike consistency. Scoop up a heaping tablespoon of the mixture; form into a ball. Flatten with your palms.

3. Flour the patties on both sides.

4. Warm oil to about ½ inch up the sides of a large skillet over medium-high heat. Cook the patties until golden brown on each side.

5. Transfer to a paper towel–lined plate until ready to serve.

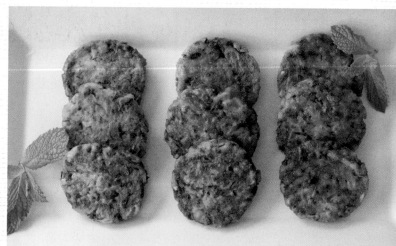

Spinach Patties

This recipe is diabetic-friendly!

3 (10-ounce) boxes frozen spinach, coarsely chopped

4 scallions, sliced

3 large eggs

1 cup bread crumbs

1 large onion, chopped

1 cup grated Romano cheese

½ cup crumbled feta cheese

½ cup minced fresh dill

Black pepper

1 cup all-purpose flour

Olive oil, for frying

EveryGirl

TIP: Serve these patties warm, with a squeeze of lemon juice.

1. Defrost the chopped spinach in a strainer set in the sink.

2. In a large bowl, combine the spinach, scallions, eggs, bread crumbs, onion, Romano and feta cheeses, dill, and pepper to taste. Using your hands, form small balls. Flatten into patties with your palms.

3. Flour the patties on both sides.

4. Warm oil to about a half inch up the sides of a large skillet over medium-high heat. Cook the patties until golden brown on each side.

5. Transfer to a paper towel–lined plate until ready to serve.

Zucchini-Almond Patties

MAKES ABOUT 25 PATTIES

This recipe is diabetic-friendly!

4 medium zucchini, shredded and squeezed of excess water
1 large egg
1 cup bread crumbs
½ cup crushed almonds
½ cup chopped fresh parsley
½ cup chopped fresh mint
4 cloves garlic, minced
Salt and black pepper
1 cup all-purpose flour
Olive oil, for frying

EveryGirl
TIP: Be sure to use unseasoned bread crumbs. It's much better to add your own seasonings.

1. In a large bowl, combine the shredded zucchini, egg, bread crumbs, almonds, parsley, mint, garlic, and salt and pepper. Scoop up a heaping tablespoon of the mixture; form into a ball. Repeat with the remaining mixture and flatten into patties with your palms.

2. Flour the patties on both sides.

3. Warm oil to about ½ inch up the sides of a large skillet over medium-high heat. Cook the patties until golden brown on each side.

4. Transfer to a paper towel–lined plate until ready to serve.

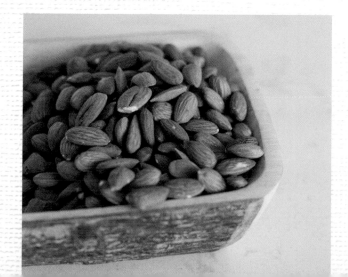

Tzatziki

SERVES 10 This recipe is diabetic-friendly and gluten-free!

3 cups Greek yogurt

1 large cucumber (the long skinny kind)

1 tablespoon salt

1 clove garlic, minced

3 tablespoons lemon juice (or juice of 1 lemon)

1 tablespoon fresh dill

2 tablespoons finely chopped fresh parsley

Black pepper

1. Strain the yogurt for a few hours or overnight in the fridge.

2. Peel the cucumber and dice. Put it in a colander and sprinkle with the salt. Cover with a plate or lid. Let it sit for 30 minutes, then drain well and blot dry with a paper towel.

3. In a food processor or blender, add the cucumber, garlic, lemon juice, dill, parsley, and a few grinds of black pepper. Process until well blended, then stir into the yogurt. Taste before adding any extra salt.

4. Place in the refrigerator for at least 2 hours before serving, for optimal taste.

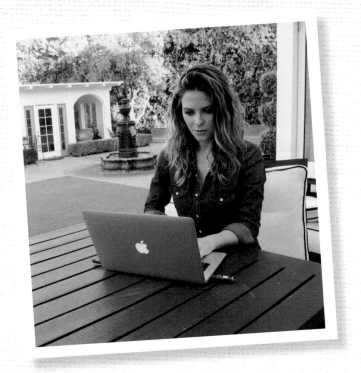

EveryGirl COOKING MOMENT

If you haven't already guessed, I'm always up for trying new things in the kitchen. We used to have some old pomegranate trees in our front yard, and one year they bloomed incredibly, leaving us with a rather plentiful crop. I felt like it would be such a waste not to do something with them. Thus I Googled "pomegranate recipes" and saw one for pomegranate ice cream. I went to work and created a healthy and tasty concoction! I know most of you don't have pomegranate trees growing in your front yards, but maybe you are craving a certain fruit or have an abundance on hand that is about to spoil. Hit Google and see what comes up—you may be surprised!

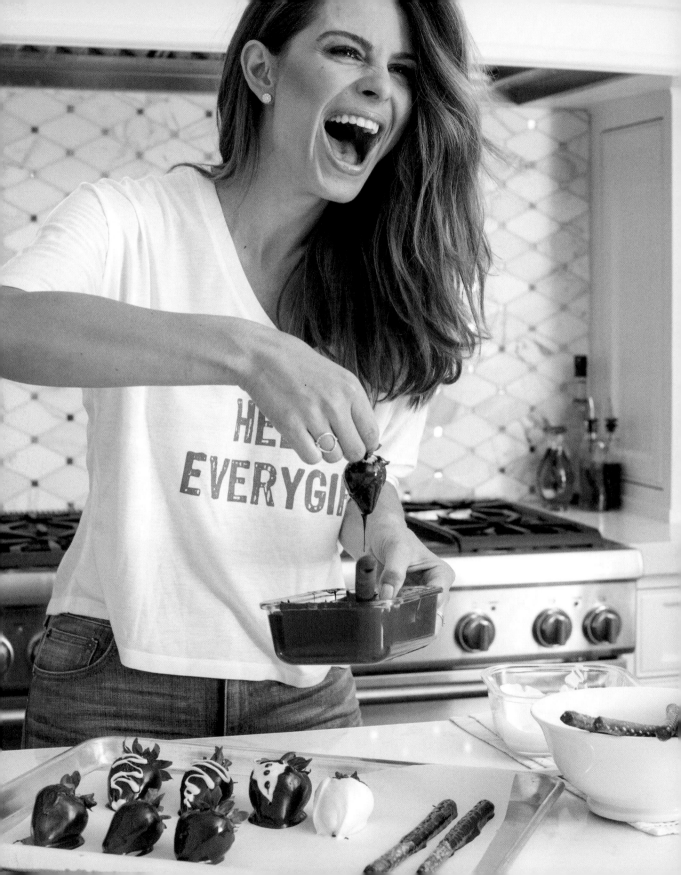

EveryGirl
DESSERTS

I tend to eat dessert most when I'm entertaining and even then I usually make so many appetizers and dinner items that there isn't much room for dessert. But who can say no to an oatmeal chocolate chip cookie? Especially when I time them perfectly to come out of the oven so people can eat them while they are warm. There are some other great desserts in *The EveryGirl's Guide to Life* as well as *The EveryGirl's Guide to Diet and Fitness* . . . including some lower-calorie, guilt-free alternatives.

Best Banana Bread

You might think of banana bread as a breakfast treat, but it also hits the spot at the end of the evening meal, so don't toss those black-peel bananas! Turn them into the moistest banana bread you will ever meet. The riper the bananas, the better the flavor.

8 tablespoons (1 stick) unsalted butter, at room temperature, plus extra for the pan

2 cups all-purpose flour, plus extra for the pan

1½ teaspoons baking soda

Pinch of salt

1 cup granulated sugar

2 large eggs

1 teaspoon vanilla extract

6 ripe bananas, mashed

1 cup chopped walnuts

1. Preheat the oven to 325°F. Butter and lightly flour a 9-inch loaf pan.

2. In a bowl, whisk the flour, baking soda, and salt until combined.

3. In a large bowl (using an electric mixer, if desired), beat the butter and sugar until combined. Beat in the eggs and vanilla, then the mashed bananas, leaving some chunky banana pieces.

4. Fold in the flour mixture just until combined. Fold in the walnuts.

5. Scoop the batter into the prepared pan. Bake for 50 minutes to 1 hour, until a toothpick inserted into the bread comes out with a few moist crumbs.

6. Transfer to a wire rack to cool for 10 minutes. Run a knife around the bread in the pan; carefully remove from the pan. Let cool completely on a wire rack.

EveryGirl

TIP: For ease in blending, make sure your butter is at room temperature. After you've dropped the sticks into the mixing bowl, use the buttery stick wrappers to grease the loaf pan.

Anytime Oatmeal Fruit Crumble

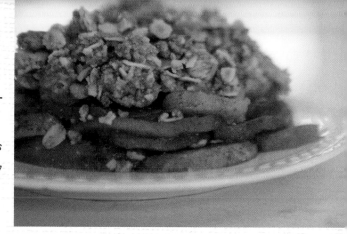

SERVES 8

Here's another dessert made up of ingredients more traditionally used at breakfast time. I say mix and match!

Fruit

4 cups thinly sliced peeled fruit, such as apples, pears, or peaches

3 tablespoons granulated sugar

½ teaspoon cinnamon

Crumble

1 cup all-purpose flour

1 cup quick or old-fashioned oats

½ cup brown sugar

½ teaspoon cinnamon

¼ teaspoon salt

8 tablespoons (1 stick) unsalted butter, melted

EveryGirl
TIP: Baking time will vary with the type of fruit used. Apples and pears take longer to cook than peaches.

EveryGirl
TIP: Add vanilla ice cream or Cool Whip on top. Yum!

1. Preheat the oven to 350°F.

2. In a large bowl, toss the sliced fruit with the 3 tablespoons sugar and ½ teaspoon cinnamon. Pour the fruit into a pie pan.

3. For the crumble: In the same bowl (no need to wash), combine the flour, oats, brown sugar, cinnamon, and salt. Fold in the melted butter until the mixture forms moist clumps.

4. Sprinkle the crumble mixture over the fruit. Bake for 45 minutes, or until the topping is golden and the fruit is bubbling.

Oatmeal Chocolate Chip Cookies with Toasted Pecans

MAKES 32 COOKIES

Guests love it when you serve these cookies fresh out of the oven—hot and melty! If you're making them for yourself, make sure to eat one that way, too (and then save the rest for later).

EveryGirl

TIP: You can make the dough a few days in advance—it will keep in the refrigerator until you are ready to bake.

EveryGirl

TIP: If you want cookies that are crisp on the outside and chewy on the inside, make sure to undercook them a little bit.

EveryGirl

TIP: If you have a food processor, make the dough in that; it will make the cookies more "fluffy."

1 cup pecans

1¾ cups all-purpose flour

1 teaspoon baking soda

1 teaspoon salt

½ teaspoon baking powder

1 cup (2 sticks) unsalted butter, cool, but not cold

1 cup brown sugar

½ cup granulated sugar

1 whole egg and 1 egg yolk

1 teaspoon pure vanilla extract

2 cups old-fashioned oats or quick oatmeal

1½ cups semisweet chocolate chips or chunks

½ cup shredded unsweetened or sweetened coconut

1. Preheat the oven to 350°F.

2. Spread the pecans in a single layer on a rimmed baking sheet. Toast for 8 minutes, or until lightly browned around the edges. Let cool; coarsely chop.

3. In a large bowl, combine the flour, baking soda, salt, and baking powder.

4. In a large bowl, with an electric mixer, cream the butter and both sugars until fluffy. Reduce the speed and add the egg and yolk, one at a time, beating well after each addition. Beat in the vanilla. Gradually add the flour mixture, beating until just incorporated.

5. Using a spatula, fold in the oats, chocolate, coconut, and toasted pecans until just combined.

6. Line baking sheets with parchment paper or nonstick liner, or lightly coat with cooking spray. Drop the dough in rounded tablespoons on the prepared sheets about 3 inches apart. Bake, one sheet at a time, for 12 to 14 minutes, until the cookies are golden around the edges, but still a little wet-looking in the middle.

7. Transfer the sheets to a wire rack and let cool for 5 minutes. Using a spatula, transfer the cookies to a rack to cool completely.

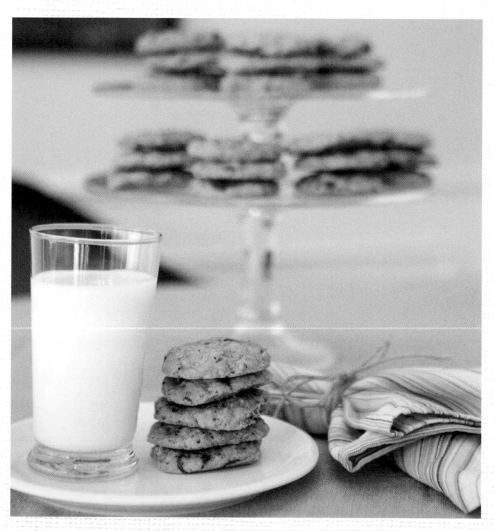

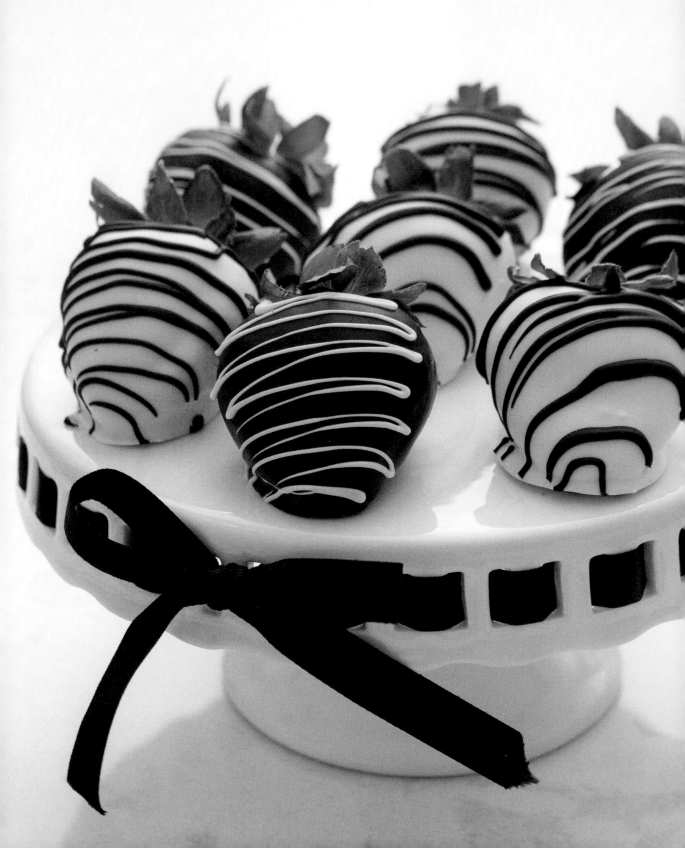

Chocolate-Covered Strawberries (or anything else that you like)

MAKES 12

You can buy chocolate-dipped strawberries perfect and pretty at the store, or you can have fun with it and make them yourself. I think the imperfect homemade version is more special! Have fun with the designs; that's the point of making them yourself. I like to try to make them look like my guests so they can try and guess which is theirs.

4 ounces dark chocolate chips

2 ounces white chocolate chips

12 strawberries

Powdered sugar

Large-grain sugar crystals, any color

1. Place the chocolate in two separate glass bowls and microwave in 30-second intervals, until melted, stirring in between intervals.

2. Holding a strawberry by the stem end, dip it in the dark chocolate, letting the excess chocolate drip back into the bowl.

3. Transfer each dipped berry onto a baking sheet lined with wax or parchment paper, and allow the chocolate to harden. As you set each berry down, slide it ½ inch to the side to prevent chocolate from clumping under the berry.

4. Drizzle the melted white chocolate back and forth over the berries. Repeat with the remaining berries. Before the chocolate sets, sprinkle one side, or the pointed ends, with powdered sugar or large-grain sugar.

EveryGirl

TIP: Make these sweet treats look professional by adding a drizzle of white chocolate or a sprinkle of sparkle sugar.

EveryGirl

TIP: This works for any fruit or even pretzels!

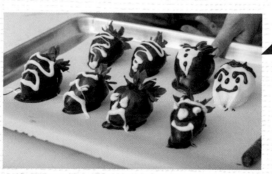

I had some fun with these. . . . Guess the celebrity's face!

Greek Yogurt Strawberry Sundae

SERVES 1

Greek yogurt is thick and rich and just like ice cream if you serve it up ice cold.

½ cup plain nonfat Greek yogurt

2 teaspoons honey

3 strawberries, sliced

2 tablespoons chopped almonds

In a serving bowl, stir the yogurt and honey. Top with the strawberries and almonds.

EveryGirl
TIP: Substitute agave for the honey or a different fruit or nut; whatever you have on hand!

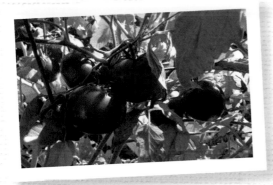
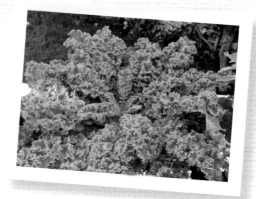

EveryGirl COOKING MOMENT

Get gardening! You don't have to have tons of space; a small 4 x 8-foot wooden or plastic box works great. Pots on your windowsill or fire escape, patio, or porch will do the trick, too. Or maybe there's a community garden nearby that you can get in on? I started with a small wooden box in our backyard, but once I got the hang of it, I invested in having a stylish red brick version constructed. Seeing the fresh vegetables in the garden inspires me to want to eat and cook better. I'm especially proud of the colors, textures, and sizes of the produce. My dad and his brothers often compete over who has the best crop annually! Check out my "odd" shaped carrot below! We had a good laugh about that one! These are all from my garden.

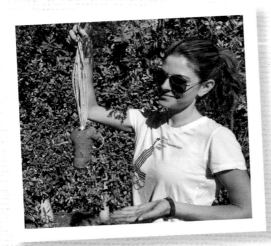
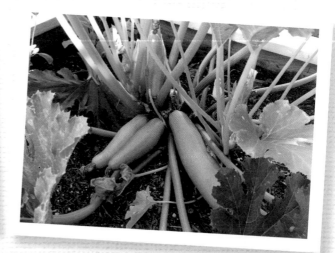

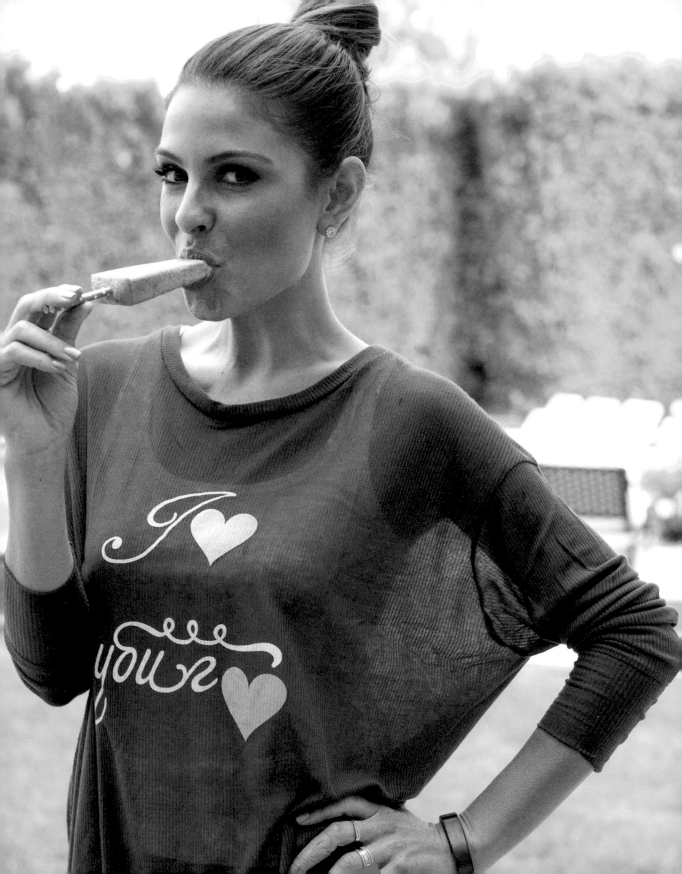

EveryGirl
GETS WELL

I can usually tell when I'm coming down with something or know when I have just pushed myself too hard and am at higher risk for a cold, the flu, or another illness. Diet can be one of the best preventatives and treatments. The right diet can boost the immune system *and* help you feel better and recover faster. I find that eating foods high in antioxidants, such as fruits and vegetables, will not only boost my overall health, but also help to protect me from viruses all year long. I also like to load up on vitamin C (like citrus fruits and strawberries) for its anti-inflammatory effects. Remember to drink lots and lots of water to flush out the toxins. I'm able to stave off and reduce bouts of illness by doing so.

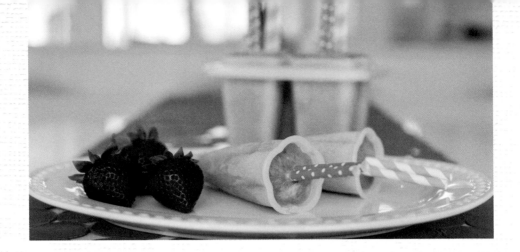

EveryGirl

TIP: To unmold the pops, run warm water briefly over the molds and gently pull on the sticks.

Strawberry Cream Pops

MAKES 5 POPS

If you are congested—especially if your cold or cough has moved to your chest—you'll want to stay away from dairy products. But if you have a sore throat or the sniffles, these soothing pops will hit the spot!

1 cup sliced fresh strawberries
1 cup plain nonfat Greek yogurt
2 tablespoons honey

I wonder if she knows they aren't real ice cream? Ha ha!

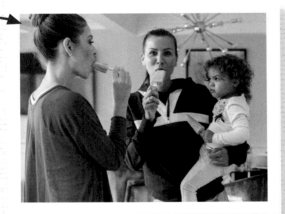

1. In a blender, combine all of the ingredients until smooth.

2. Pour into 3-ounce ice pop molds, leaving some room at the top for expansion.

3. Insert ice pop sticks; freeze for 4 hours, or until solid.

Soothing Fresh Ginger Tea

SERVES 1

Fresh ginger tea couldn't be easier, or more soothing on a sore throat. Ginger is also thought to be helpful for nausea.

    4 thin slices fresh ginger
    3 leaves fresh mint
    1 tablespoon fresh lemon juice
    1 tablespoon agave or honey
    Boiling water, as desired

1. In a large cup, combine the ginger, mint, juice, and honey.

2. Add boiling water; let steep 10 minutes.

3. Using a slotted spoon, lift out the ginger and mint.

Chicken Orzo Soup

SERVES 4   This recipe is diabetic-friendly! **D**

Nothing says "Get better soon" better than this chicken orzo soup! It's the thing I crave when I'm feeling a little under the weather.

¼ cup olive oil

1 small onion, chopped

2 carrots, peeled and sliced

2 stalks celery, sliced

2 cloves garlic, chopped

¾ pound boneless, skinless chicken breast halves

1 dried bay leaf

Salt and black pepper

4 cups reduced-sodium chicken broth

4 ounces (½ cup) orzo or other small pasta

1. Warm 2 teaspoons of the oil in a large pot over medium heat. Cook the onion, carrots, and celery, stirring occasionally, until they are softened, about 8 minutes.

2. Stir in the garlic; cook for 30 seconds, stirring.

3. Clear a space in the middle of the pan; add the remaining 2 teaspoons oil and the chicken. Cook for 3 minutes per side, until golden.

4. Add the bay leaf and season with salt and pepper. Pour in half the broth (about 2 cups). Bring to a simmer; reduce the heat to medium-low. Simmer for 25 minutes.

5. Using tongs, transfer the chicken to a cutting board and shred. Return to the soup, along with the remaining broth.

6. Bring to a simmer, and add the orzo. Cook for 5 minutes, or until the pasta is just al dente. Season with salt and pepper.

EveryGirl

TIP: The length of the final cooking time depends on the size of the pasta used. Remember that the pasta will continue to cook after you've taken the pot off the heat. So remove the pot from the burner when the pasta is still al dente.

EveryGirl

TIP: There's no need to thaw frozen peas before adding them to the soup.

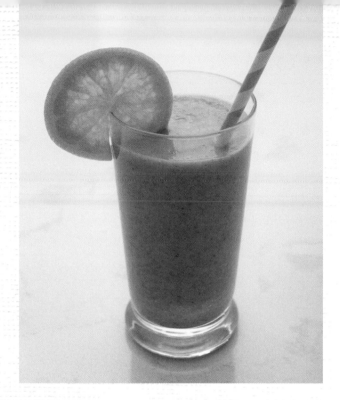

EveryGirl

TIP: Use fresh, frozen, or canned pineapple. Stay away from the type that's packed in syrup.

Immunity-Boosting Cold-Kicking Smoothie

SERVES 2

The name of this recipe says it all! Add lots of ice if you have a sore throat.

- 1½ cups pineapple chunks
- 1 cup chopped fresh kale
- 1 frozen banana, cut into chunks
- ½ cup orange juice
- 1 full drop echinacea liquid
- ½ cup ice chips

1. In a blender or food processor, process the pineapple chunks, kale, banana chunks, orange juice, echinacea, and ice chips until blended.

2. Add additional ice chips to achieve the desired consistency.

Maria's Miracle Mix

SERVES 1

When I'm coming down with something, here's one of my go-to cures.

Mix a few drops of Thieves oil, oil of oregano, and echinacea in a shot of water. I take this concoction once a day the second I start feeling a little sick, and it works every time!

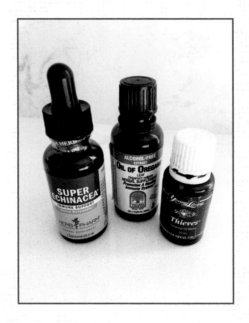

EveryGirl COOKING MOMENT

In Hollywood, Mom and I don't just cook for bosses, coworkers, and kitchen icons—we make plates for many or most of the talk shows I appear on. Mom has made dishes and desserts for Howard Stern, the *Today* show team, Conan, Jimmy Kimmel, *GMA*, and many other shows. It's a great way to say thanks for having me on. They appreciate the gesture and so do their crews. When I make return appearances, many will make specific requests that we happily fulfill! We have also sent thank-you dessert baskets to those who have been supportive of me and my career throughout the years. We take steps to make the baskets as beautiful as possible, too. People love the thought and effort more than a purchased gift.

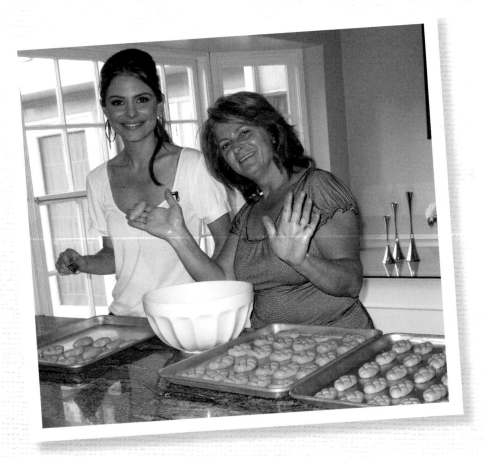

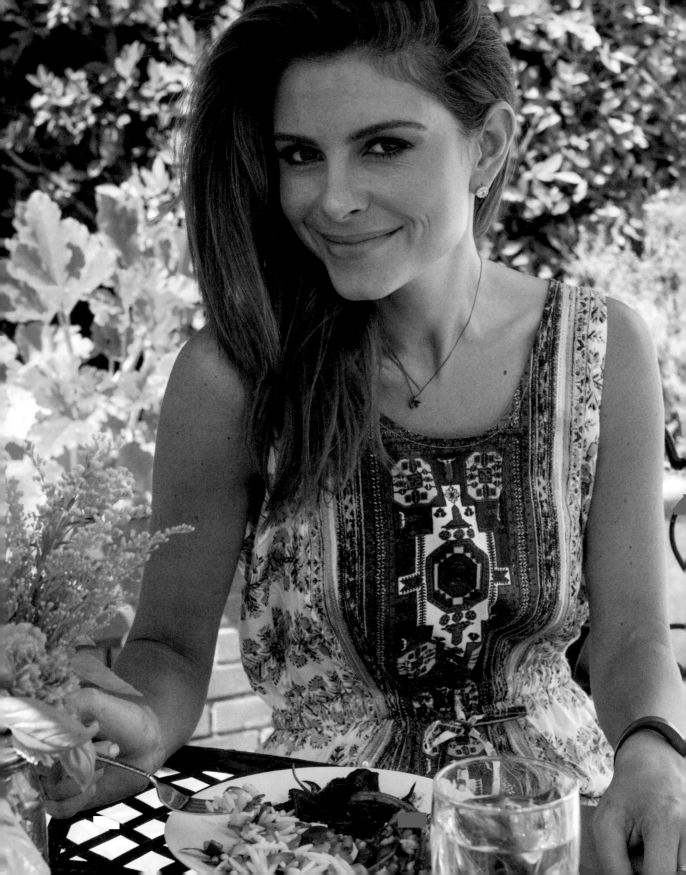

EveryGirl

GO-TO DRESSINGS

There's no need to reach for a bottled (and often preservative-filled) salad dressing when you can make one of these delicious dressings quickly at home. Use them for green or grain salads or vegetable dishes. Another bonus? These dressings will keep for days in your refrigerator. I like to make them in an empty jam jar. Once all the ingredients are in the jar, I screw on the lid and give the jar a vigorous shake.

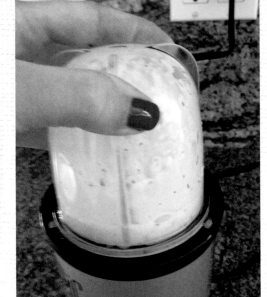

I love creamy dressings, but store-bought ones usually have sugar added, which defeats the purpose of having a clean, healthy salad. I use a Magic Bullet to blend creamier dressings of my own. Having a garden, I can mix in my own fresh herbs and spices, too. Anyone can grow herbs and spices in a small pot. I'm super obsessed with vertical gardens, too. If you haven't seen one, check them out online; you can put one just about anywhere!

EveryGirl

TIP: You can easily store the leftover dressing in a jar or bottle in your fridge.

Maria's Greek Vinaigrette

MAKES ABOUT ½ CUP   This recipe is diabetic-friendly and gluten-free!

EveryGirl

TIP: Always use extra-virgin olive oil for dressings and uncooked dishes. You can use the milder, less expensive regular-press olive oil for cooking.

3 tablespoons extra-virgin olive oil

2 tablespoons red or white wine vinegar

2 tablespoons chopped fresh parsley

1 tablespoon fresh lemon juice

½ teaspoon chopped fresh oregano

½ teaspoon salt

¼ teaspoon black pepper

In a bowl or measuring cup, whisk together the olive oil, vinegar, parsley, lemon juice, oregano, salt, and black pepper until combined.

Greek Feta/Lemon Dressing

MAKES ABOUT ¾ CUP   This recipe is diabetic-friendly and gluten-free!

½ cup extra-virgin olive oil
¼ cup fresh lemon juice
2 cloves garlic, minced
¼ teaspoon salt
1 tablespoon crumbled feta cheese

In a bowl or measuring cup, whisk together the olive oil, lemon juice, garlic, salt, and feta cheese until combined.

EveryGirl

TIP: This recipe makes a lot of dressing, enough for several salads. It will keep for several days in the fridge. It will thicken when cold, so let it sit out on the counter to warm up, then give it a good stir before adding to your salad.

Oil and Lemon Dressing

MAKES ABOUT ⅔ CUP   This recipe is diabetic-friendly and gluten-free!

½ cup extra-virgin olive oil
3 tablespoons fresh lemon juice
2 teaspoons chopped fresh oregano
½ teaspoon salt
¼ teaspoon black pepper

In a bowl or measuring cup, whisk together the olive oil, lemon juice, oregano, salt, and pepper until combined.

EveryGirl

TIP: If you don't have, or don't care for, oregano, substitute any chopped fresh herb. Or use no herb at all!

EveryGirl

TIP: I like to add other herbs from my garden like basil, rosemary, scallions, and even garlic to switch it up. Don't be afraid to play around a little; that's how I learned, too.

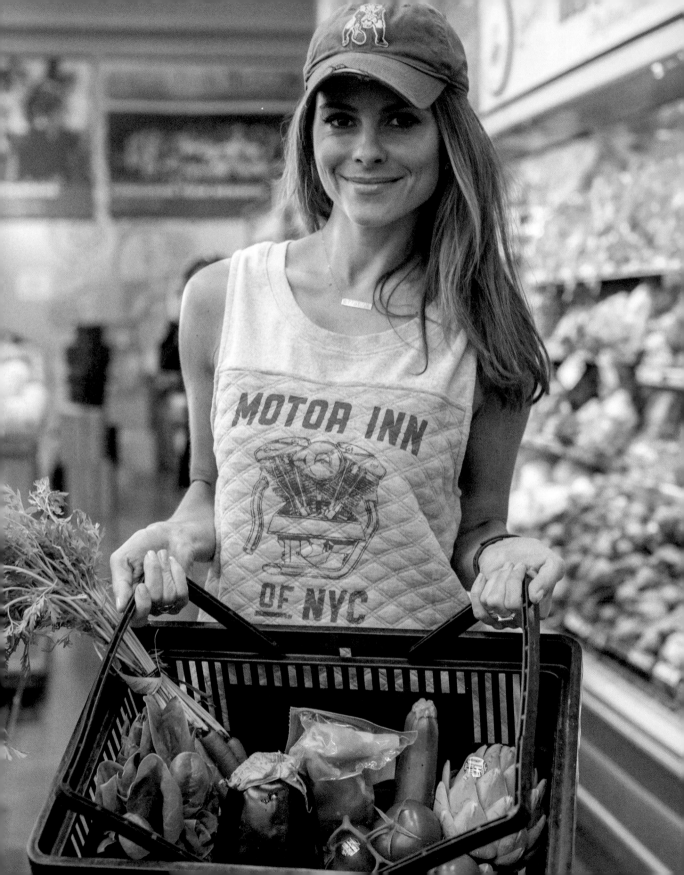

Everygirl

COOKS WITH
10 INGREDIENTS

This is the bonus section designed specifically for women like me who *really* want and need to keep it simple. And for those women who get home and want to make a recipe and then realize they lack all the key ingredients in the fridge and pantry. They can either go to the supermarket and get the items (ugh, who wants to do that when you're probably already starving?) or abandon the idea of cooking and go out to eat. This happens to me all the time and 99 out of 100 times I end up going out to eat. That's why I came up with the idea to make one grocery list with ten ingredients to make different meals for one week. The idea is that you can have 4 different shopping lists on your phone, ready to go when you're at the store, and you know what to buy for the next week to make 5 delicious meals. Keep in mind, to do so, you must have your previously listed key pantry items in stock. Also, remember to buy each week according to how many nights you want to cook and for how many people. For example, if this week you are only cooking two nights, buy only enough ingredients for two nights' worth of meals.

Be sure to have your cabinets stocked with EveryGirl Pantry Basics (page 279).

GROUP 1

1. Chicken tenders
2. Eggs
3. Feta cheese
4. Ground beef
5. Onions
6. Potatoes
7. Shrimp
8. Spinach
9. Tomatoes
10. Zucchini

WEEK MENU

DAY 1
Spicy Shrimp with Spaghetti *Serves 4, page 230*

DAY 2
Baked Stuffed Tomatoes with Feta *Serves 4, page 232*

DAY 3
Baked Chicken and Potatoes *Serves 2, page 233*

DAY 4
Spinach-Stuffed Potatoes with Melted Cheese *Serves 2, page 234*

DAY 5
Grilled Zucchini and Shrimp with Feta *Serves 2, page 235*

SHOPPING LIST GROUP 1

BUY THESE ITEMS AT THE GROCERY STORE:

1 pound feta cheese

6 large beefsteak tomatoes

6 chicken tenders

6 large eggs

1 pound ground beef

2 medium onions

2 large and 4 small russet potatoes

2 bags frozen shrimp (pound-size, peeled and deveined)

1 small bag spinach leaves

3 zucchini

All of these ingredients will yield five recipes. If you aren't cooking five days this week, reduce ingredients accordingly.

CHECK YOUR PANTRY FOR:

spaghetti	red pepper flakes
dried parsley	fresh garlic
quinoa or rice	dried oregano
dried basil	lemon juice
olive oil	salt and pepper

EveryGirl
TIP: When you buy meat for an entire week, make sure you freeze the packages you don't need until later on, so they don't go bad.

EveryGirl
TIP: You only need one egg for this week, but then you have extra for a yummy omelet for breakfast, too.

Day 1

EveryGirl

TIP: Frozen shrimp is already peeled and deveined. Let it thaw overnight in the fridge. For faster thawing, take the shrimp out of the package, put in a bowl of cold water, and let a trickle of cold water run into the bowl while excess water goes down the drain. The shrimp should be ready to cook in 15 minutes.

EveryGirl

TIP: Adjust the amount of pepper flakes depending on how spicy you want the dish.

EveryGirl

TIP: If it's not tomato season and your tomatoes aren't juicy, you may want to add some water during the cooking time to make the sauce saucier.

Spicy Shrimp with Spaghetti

SERVES 4   (D if whole-wheat; GF if GF spaghetti)

½ pound spaghetti (regular, whole-grain, or gluten-free)

2 tablespoons olive oil

2 large tomatoes, diced

3 cloves garlic, chopped

½ teaspoon red pepper flakes, or as desired

1 pound frozen medium shrimp, thawed, peeled, and deveined

1 tablespoon dried basil

¼ cup dried parsley

Salt and black pepper

1. Cook the pasta according to the package directions; drain.

2. Warm the oil in a large skillet over medium heat. Add the tomatoes, garlic, and pepper flakes, mashing the tomatoes against the side of the skillet. Increase the heat to medium-high and simmer, stirring, for 5 minutes, or until the mixture has thickened.

3. Add the shrimp; cook for 4 minutes, stirring and turning the shrimp to coat with the sauce.

4. Remove from the heat; stir in the drained pasta, the basil, and the parsley. Season with salt and pepper to taste.

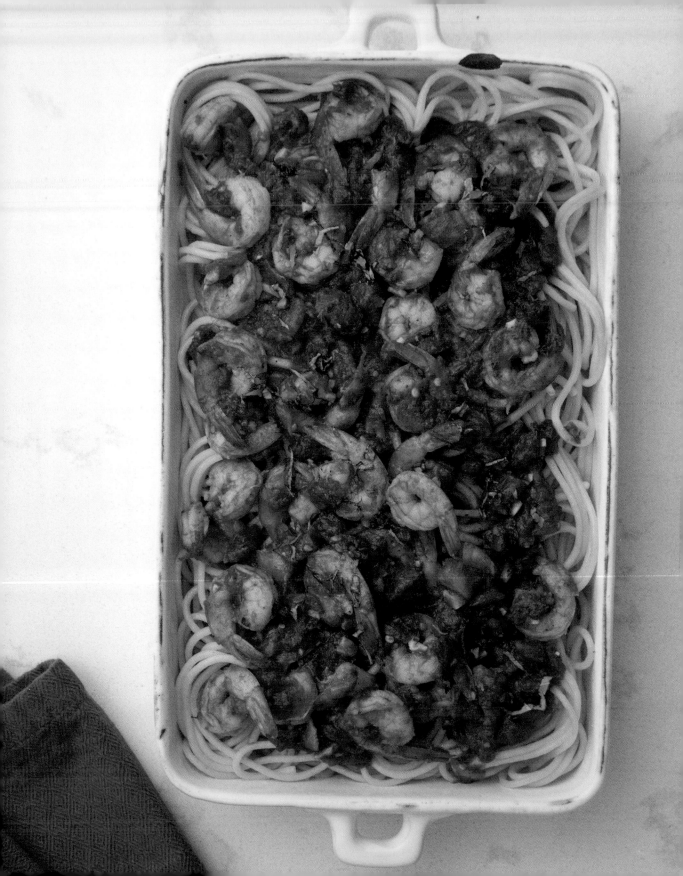

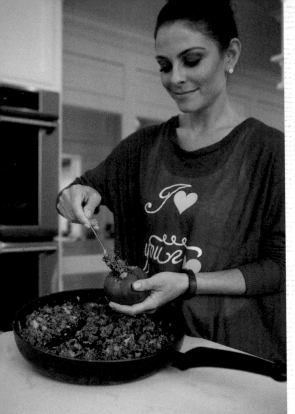

Day 2

Baked Stuffed Tomatoes with Feta

SERVES 4   (D if brown rice or quinoa) **D** **GF**

4 large beefsteak tomatoes
2 tablespoons olive oil
1 medium onion, diced
8 ounces ground beef
2 cloves garlic, chopped
Salt and black pepper
¼ cup dried parsley
½ cup cooked quinoa or brown or white rice
¼ cup feta, crumbled

1. Preheat the oven to 350°F.

2. Scoop out the flesh of the tomatoes leaving a border around the edges; place the insides in a bowl and set aside. Set the hollowed tomatoes on a rimmed baking sheet.

3. Warm the oil in a medium skillet over medium heat. Cook the onion for 5 minutes, or until softened, stirring.

4. Add the beef, the insides of the tomatoes, and the garlic, and season with salt and pepper to taste. Cook for 8 minutes, or until the beef is browned, stirring often. Stir in the parsley and quinoa.

5. Fill the tomatoes with the mixture and sprinkle with the feta on top. Bake for 25 minutes, or until warmed through.

EveryGirl
TIP: The original Greek recipe uses rice. You can substitute cooked quinoa or brown rice, if you prefer.

Day 3

Baked Chicken and Potatoes

SERVES 2   **GF**

6 chicken tenders

4 small potatoes, cut into ½-inch wedges

¼ cup olive oil

2 tablespoons lemon juice

1 tablespoon dried oregano

Salt and black pepper

1. Preheat the oven to 350°F.

2. In a 9 x 13-inch baking pan, combine the chicken, potatoes, oil, lemon juice, oregano, and salt and pepper to taste; toss to coat.

3. Bake, uncovered, for 25 minutes, or until the chicken and potatoes are cooked through. Stir a couple of times during baking.

EveryGirl
TIP: Don't forget to stir during the cooking time, to assure delicious crusty edges on the chicken and potatoes.

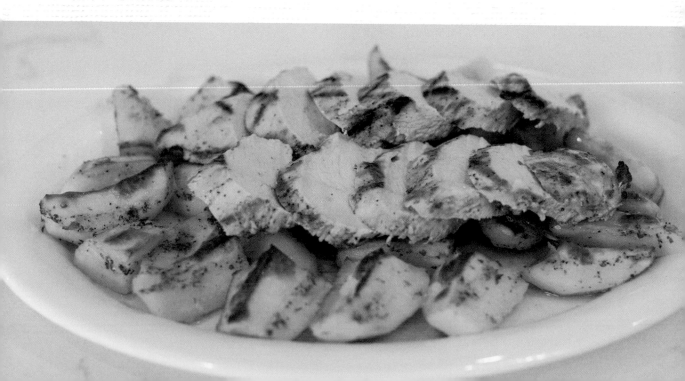

Day 4

Spinach-Stuffed Potatoes with Melted Cheese

SERVES 2

2 large russet potatoes

3 teaspoons olive oil

1 large egg

1 teaspoon garlic powder

1 onion, finely chopped

1 cup chopped spinach leaves

Salt and black pepper

¼ cup crumbled feta cheese

1. Preheat the oven to 350°F.

2. Rub the potato skins with 1 teaspoon of the oil. Place the potatoes on a plate and microwave on high for 12 minutes, rotating the potatoes halfway through cooking. Slice the potatoes in half horizontally and place on a baking sheet.

3. Scoop out the flesh of the potatoes and place in a bowl. Stir in the remaining 2 teaspoons oil, the egg, garlic powder, onion, and spinach, and salt and pepper to taste.

4. Scoop the filling into the potatoes; sprinkle with the feta cheese, and bake for about 20 minutes, until the cheese melts.

EveryGirl

TIP: Partially cooking the potatoes in the microwave means this satisfying dish can be on the table in about a half hour. You can use either sweet or white potatoes—or one of each!

Day 5

Grilled Zucchini and Shrimp with Feta

SERVES 2

2 tablespoons olive oil
1 tablespoon minced garlic
1 tablespoon lemon juice
1 tablespoon dried parsley
Salt and black pepper
3 zucchini, unpeeled, cut on the diagonal into long ½-inch-thick slices
8 to 10 frozen medium shrimp, thawed, peeled, and deveined
¼ cup crumbled feta cheese

1. Coat a grill rack or grill pan with nonstick cooking spray or rub with an oil-soaked paper towel. Preheat the grill to medium.

2. In a large shallow dish, combine the oil, garlic, lemon juice, parsley, and salt and pepper to taste. Add the zucchini slices; turn to coat on both sides.

3. Place the zucchini on the grill; cook for 5 minutes per side, or until lightly browned and cooked through.

4. Meanwhile, toss the shrimp with the marinade remaining in the dish. Grill the shrimp for 2 minutes per side, until just cooked.

5. On a platter, toss the zucchini and shrimp with the feta. Serve warm or at room temperature.

EveryGirl
TIP: Grilling times will vary greatly depending on the type of grill used, the air temperature, and the wind conditions. Use these cooking times as guidelines, and take the zucchini off the grill when it is softened, but not mushy, with pretty grill marks.

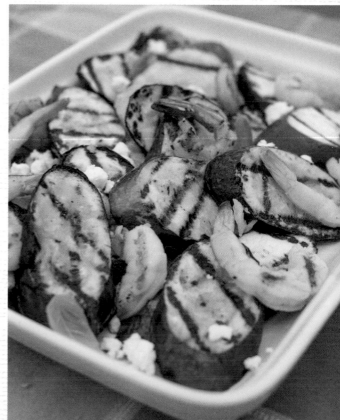

GROUP 2

1. Carrots
2. Celery
3. Chicken breast
4. Green beans
5. Peas

6. Red onion
7. Red bell peppers
8. Red potatoes
9. White beans
10. Cheddar cheese

WEEK MENU

DAY 1
White Bean Soup *Serves 2, page 239*

DAY 2
Pan-Roasted Chicken and Green Bean Bake *Serves 3 or 4, page 240*

DAY 3
White Bean and Brown Rice Pilaf *Serves 3 or 4, page 241*

DAY 4
Lemon Chicken Salad *Serves 2, page 242*

DAY 5
Chicken with Peppers and Onions *Serves 4, page 243*

SHOPPING LIST GROUP 2

3 carrots

4 boneless, skinless chicken breast halves and 4 bone-in, skinless chicken breast halves

10 ounces fresh green beans

5 medium onions

1 small bag frozen peas

3 red bell peppers

3 small red potatoes

2 stalks celery

2 cans white beans (15 ounces each)

1 small bag shredded Cheddar cheese

CHECK YOUR PANTRY FOR:

tomato sauce	dried parsley
brown rice	lemon juice
chicken broth, reduced-sodium	Parmesan cheese
	olive oil
fresh garlic	salt and pepper

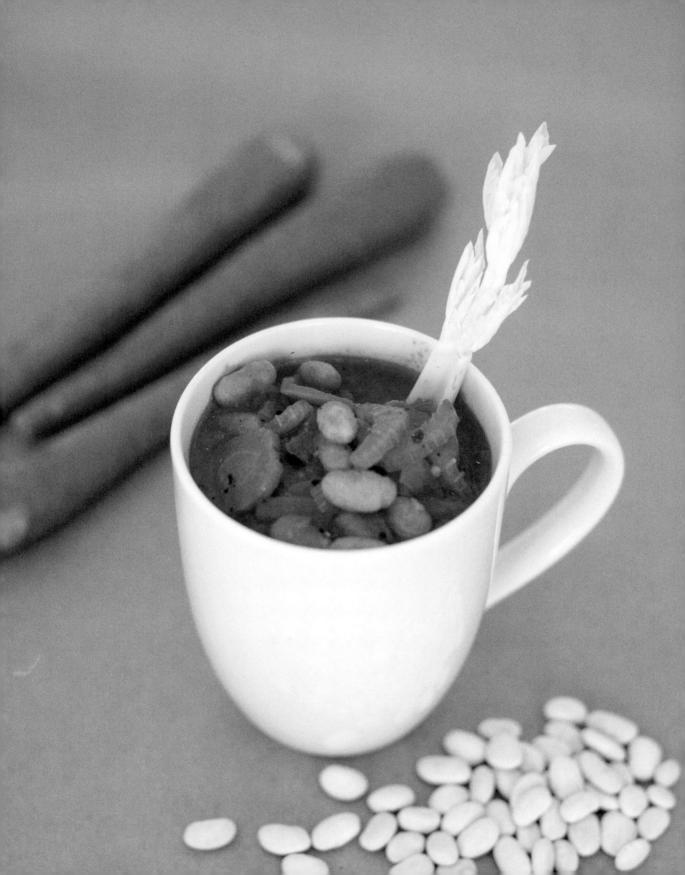

Day 1

White Bean Soup

SERVES 2

1 can (14½ ounces) white kidney beans, drained and rinsed

1 can (8 ounces) tomato sauce

2 tablespoons olive oil

1 onion, chopped

1 stalk celery, sliced

1 carrot, peeled and sliced

Salt and black pepper, to taste

1. Combine all of the ingredients and 2 cups water in a medium saucepan over medium-high heat.

2. Simmer for 15 to 20 minutes, stirring occasionally. Add water, if needed, for the desired consistency.

EveryGirl
TIP: This simple soup tastes even better the next day!

EveryGirl
TIP: Add more water if you want a thinner soup.

Day 2

Pan-Roasted Chicken and Green Bean Bake

SERVES 3 OR 4

¼ cup olive oil

1 medium onion, diced

1 stalk celery, diced

10 ounces green beans, trimmed and halved

4 bone-in, skinless chicken breast halves (about 2 pounds)

Salt and black pepper

¾ cup reduced-sodium chicken broth

½ cup shredded Cheddar cheese

1. Warm the oil in a large cast-iron or other heavy ovenproof skillet over medium heat. Add the onion, celery, and green beans; cook for 5 minutes, stirring. Remove the vegetables and set aside.

2. Place the chicken in the center of the skillet, season with salt and pepper to taste, add the broth and cook for about 20 minutes, turning occasionally, until the chicken is golden and cooked through.

3. Remove the chicken to a platter; place the skillet over medium-high heat and return the vegetables to the pan and simmer for 2 minutes to reduce the liquid in the pan. Pour the sauce around the chicken on the platter.

4. Add the cheese on top of the hot vegetables until melted. Serve with the chicken.

Day 3

White Bean and Brown Rice Pilaf

SERVES 3 OR 4   (GF- if rice or GF pasta)

1 cup brown rice
2 tablespoons olive oil
1 medium onion, diced
2 medium carrots, diced
3 cloves garlic, chopped
1 can (15 ounces) white beans, drained and rinsed
1 can (7 ounces) tomato sauce
Salt and black pepper
½ cup frozen peas
½ cup grated Parmesan cheese

EveryGirl
TIP: Use any cooked grain or pasta in this hearty, homey, vegetarian dish. You can please meat lovers by stirring in some cooked ground beef, turkey, or sausage with the beans.

1. Preheat the oven to 375°F.

2. In a medium saucepan, bring the rice and 2½ cups of water to a boil over high heat. When boiling, reduce the heat to low and simmer, covered, for 20 minutes.

3. Warm the oil in a large, heavy ovenproof skillet over medium heat. Add the onion, carrots, and garlic; cook for 10 minutes, stirring.

4. Stir in the beans, tomato sauce, rice, and 1 cup water. Season with salt and pepper to taste and bring to a simmer. Transfer to the oven and cook for 15 minutes, or until warmed through and the rice is tender.

5. Increase the oven temperature to broil. Stir in the peas and top with the cheese. Broil for 1 minute, or until the cheese melts.

Day 4

Lemon Chicken Salad

SERVES 2   (D- if whole wheat pita, GF if no pita)

2 boneless, skinless chicken breast halves
¼ cup olive oil
2 tablespoons lemon juice
½ cup diced celery
½ cup diced red bell pepper
2 tablespoons diced red onion
2 tablespoons dried parsley
Salt and black pepper

EveryGirl

TIP: Make this super-quick salad your own by using whatever herb you like best. Serve the salad on a bed of lettuce or stuffed into a pita.

1. Place the chicken in a medium saucepan and cover with water by at least 1 inch; bring to a boil over medium-high heat.

2. Reduce the heat to a simmer, cover, and cook for 10 to 12 minutes, until the chicken is cooked through.

3. Remove the chicken from the liquid and dice or shred.

4. In a medium serving bowl, whisk the oil and lemon juice. Fold in the chicken, celery, red bell pepper, onion, and parsley. Season with salt and pepper to taste.

Day 5

Chicken with Peppers and Onions

SERVES 4

¼ cup olive oil

2 boneless, skinless chicken breast halves, cut into thick slices

Salt and black pepper

3 small red potatoes, diced

2 medium onions, thinly sliced

½ cup diced celery

1½ red bell peppers, diced

1 can (8 ounces) tomato sauce

3 cloves garlic, chopped

3 tablespoons dried parsley

1. Warm the oil in a large cast-iron or heavy ovenproof skillet over medium-high heat.

2. Season the chicken with salt and pepper. Cook the chicken, potatoes, onions, celery, and red peppers until the chicken is lightly browned, stirring occasionally.

3. Add the tomato sauce, garlic, and parsley. Reduce the heat to medium-low and cook until the potatoes are cooked through.

EveryGirl
TIP: There are two ways to ensure chicken is cooked through. Either cut into the breast to make sure the juices are clear or use an instant-read thermometer. The thermometer should register 165 degrees.

GROUP 3

1. Chicken breast
2. Zucchini
3. Tomatoes
4. Red potatoes
5. Onions

6. Eggs
7. Milk
8. Ground beef
9. Sweet potatoes
10. Fettuccine

WEEK MENU

DAY 1
Tourlou *Serves 6, page 246*

DAY 2
Chicken with Rosemary-Roasted Red Potatoes *Serves 2, page 247*

DAY 3
Skillet Chicken, Onion, and Rice *Serves 2, page 248*

DAY 4
Avgolemono Soup *Serves 6, page 249*

DAY 5
Fettuccine with Meatballs *Serves 6, page 250*

SHOPPING LIST GROUP 3

6 boneless, skinless chicken breast halves

6 large eggs

1 pound fresh or dried fettuccine

2 pounds lean ground beef

4 medium onions

2 pounds red potatoes

1 tablespoon dried rosemary

5 cans (7 ounces) tomato sauce

3 large tomatoes

2 zucchini

2 sweet potatoes

1 gallon low-fat milk

CHECK YOUR PANTRY FOR:

tomato sauce	fresh garlic
dried basil	lemon juice
bread crumbs	olive oil
brown or white rice	Parmesan cheese
chicken broth, reduced-sodium	dried parsley
	red pepper flakes
dried rosemary	salt and black pepper

Day 1

Tourlou

SERVES 6

EveryGirl
TIP: Serve this hearty meal directly from the rustic cast-iron skillet.

EveryGirl
TIP: If the mixture seems to be drying out during cooking, drizzle in some water.

¼ cup olive oil

3 cloves garlic, chopped

1 teaspoon parsley powder

1 teaspoon dried basil

6 red potatoes, thinly sliced

2 zucchini, thickly sliced

1 medium onion, cut into thin half-moons

2 sweet potatoes, thickly sliced

3 large ripe tomatoes, thickly sliced

1 can (8 ounces) tomato sauce

Salt and black pepper

1. Preheat the oven to 400°F.

2. Spread 2 tablespoons of the oil in a large cast-iron skillet.

3. In a small bowl, combine the garlic, parsley powder, and basil. Layer the veggies in the prepared pan in the following order: potatoes, zucchini, onion, sweet potatoes, and tomatoes. Sprinkle some of the garlic-herb mixture in between each layer. Pour the tomato sauce evenly over the vegetables in the pan.

4. Evenly drizzle with the remaining 2 tablespoons oil and season with salt and pepper to taste.

5. Bake, uncovered, for 45 minutes, or until the potatoes are tender.

Day 2

Chicken with Rosemary-Roasted Red Potatoes

SERVES 2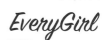

- 2 boneless, skinless chicken breast halves
- 1 pound medium red potatoes, cut into 1-inch wedges
- 2 tablespoons olive oil
- 2 tablespoons lemon juice
- 1 clove garlic, chopped
- 1 tablespoon dried rosemary
- Pinch of red pepper flakes
- Salt and black pepper

1. Preheat the oven to 375°F. Place the oven rack in the lower third of the oven.

2. Spread the chicken and potatoes on a large rimmed baking sheet. Drizzle with the oil, lemon juice, garlic, rosemary, and red pepper flakes, and season with salt and pepper to taste. Roast for 35 minutes, or until the potatoes are tender and the chicken is cooked through.

3. Turn the potatoes a few times to brown all sides.

4. Slice the chicken breasts on the diagonal; serve with the potatoes.

EveryGirl
TIP: Fresh herbs are always the best choice, but not always available. If you substitute dried herbs, remember they are stronger, so you should use less. Round out the meal with a crisp green salad.

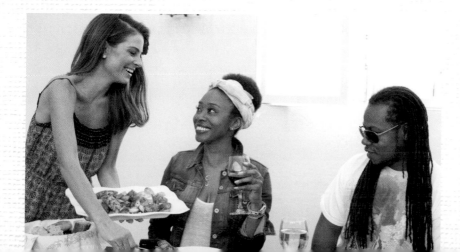

Day 3

Skillet Chicken, Onion, and Rice

SERVES 2

¼ cup olive oil

2 boneless, skinless chicken breast halves

1 medium onion, chopped

2 cloves garlic, chopped

Salt and black pepper

¾ cup reduced-sodium chicken broth

1 cup cooked brown rice

EveryGirl
TIP: Cooking the chicken in the broth makes it super-moist.

1. Warm the oil in a large nonstick skillet over medium heat. Add the chicken; cook until browned on all sides.

2. Add the onion and garlic, and season with salt and pepper; cook for 4 minutes, stirring.

3. Add the broth; cook for 5 minutes, or until mostly absorbed.

4. Mound the rice on a platter; top with the chicken and sauce.

Day 4

Avgolemono Soup

SERVES 6   (D if brown rice, GF)

2 tablespoons olive oil

1 medium onion, chopped

2 boneless, skinless chicken breast halves, cut into ½-inch chunks

Salt

4 cups (32 ounces) reduced-sodium chicken broth

1 cup cooked brown or white rice

2 large eggs

3 tablespoons lemon juice

1. Warm the oil in a large pot over medium heat. Add the onion; cook for 5 minutes or until softened, stirring.

2. Add the chicken; sprinkle with salt to taste and cook for 2 minutes, stirring. Pour in the chicken broth, rice, and 1 cup water; simmer for 1 minute.

3. In a medium bowl, whisk the eggs and lemon juice until frothy. Whisking constantly, slowly pour in a spoonful of the hot broth from the soup pot. Add 2 more spoonfuls, whisking.

4. Remove the soup from the heat; slowly pour the hot egg-lemon mixture into the soup, whisking. Serve hot.

EveryGirl

TIP: The egg-lemon mixture is a traditional finishing sauce used in many Greek dishes. Here it thickens the soup and adds a creamy texture. But don't add it all at once. Instead, follow the directions and first temper it with some of the warm soup broth.

Day 5

Fettuccine with Meatballs

SERVES 6

EveryGirl

TIP: These savory meatballs are delicious on their own—no pasta needed. But to feed a family or make a feast, toss with a pound of pasta and prepare to be worshipped!

EveryGirl

TIP: For the lightest meatballs, roll up your sleeves and mix the meat with your hands.

1 cup bread crumbs
½ cup low-fat milk
2 pounds lean ground beef
2 tablespoons dried parsley
1 egg, beaten
Salt and black pepper
3 tablespoons olive oil (divided, you'll see why)
1 tablespoon chopped onion
2 cloves garlic, chopped
32 ounces tomato sauce
1 pound fettuccine (fresh or dried)
Shredded Parmesan cheese, for garnish

1. In a small bowl, combine the bread crumbs and milk; stir to coat the crumbs.

2. In a large bowl, combine the beef, wet bread crumbs, parsley, beaten egg, and salt and pepper to taste. Form 14 to 16 two-inch meatballs.

3. Warm 2 tablespoons of the oil in a large, heavy skillet over medium heat until hot. Working in batches, brown the meatballs on all sides. Remove to a paper towel–lined plate.

4. Warm the remaining 1 tablespoon oil in the same skillet over medium heat. Cook the onion and garlic for 5 minutes, or until softened, stirring.

5. Add the tomato sauce and cook for 15 minutes, stirring. Gently lower the meatballs into the sauce and bring to a simmer. Reduce the heat to low, cover the pan, and simmer for 25 minutes, or until the meatballs are cooked through.

6. Using a wooden spoon, gently roll the meatballs during the cooking time so all sides are coated with the sauce.

7. Meanwhile, cook the pasta according to the package directions. Drain. In a large bowl, toss the pasta with the meatballs and sauce. Garnish with Parmesan, if desired.

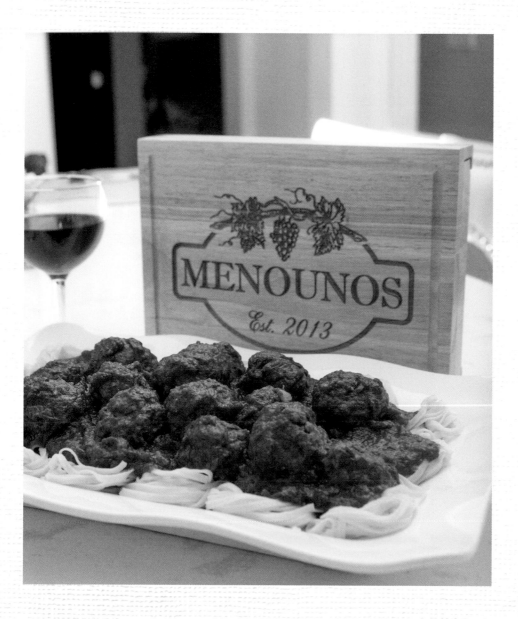

GROUP 4

1. Lentils
2. Eggs
3. Ground beef
4. Onions
5. Potatoes

6. Chicken breast
7. Spinach
8. Milk
9. Butter
10. Corn

WEEK MENU

DAY 1

Sunday Meat Loaf and Mashed Potatoes *Serves 4, page 254*

DAY 2

Speedy Spaghetti with Meat Sauce *Serves 4, page 256*

DAY 3

Greek Lentil Salad with Lemon Dressing *Serves 4, page 257*

DAY 4

Lentil Soup *Serves 4, page 259*

DAY 5

Grilled Lemon Chicken with Creamed Spinach Mashed Potatoes
Serves 4, page 260

SHOPPING LIST GROUP 4

BUY THESE ITEMS AT THE GROCERY STORE:

1 stick unsalted butter

4 boneless, skinless chicken breast halves

6 large eggs

2 pounds lean ground beef

2 pounds lentils

1 gallon low-fat milk

6 medium onions

3 medium russet potatoes

1 box fresh baby spinach

1 small bag frozen corn

CHECK YOUR PANTRY FOR:

tomato sauce	dried oregano
dried bay leaves	dried parsley
bread crumbs	dried rosemary
fresh garlic	salt and black pepper
lemon juice	spaghetti
olive oil	vinegar (red or white)

Day 1

Sunday Meat Loaf and Mashed Potatoes

SERVES 4

Meat Loaf

2 tablespoons olive oil

1 large egg, beaten

1 tablespoon chopped onion

Worcestershire sauce (as desired)

1 clove garlic, chopped

2 tablespoons dried parsley

Salt and black pepper

1 pound ground beef

½ cup corn

½ cup bread crumbs

Mashed Potatoes

1½ pounds russet potatoes, peeled and cut into large dice

4 tablespoons (½ stick) unsalted butter, cut into chunks

½ cup low-fat milk

Salt and black pepper

1. Preheat the oven to 375°F.

2. In a large bowl, whisk the oil, egg, onion, Worcestershire sauce, garlic, parsley, and salt and pepper to taste.

3. Add the beef, corn, and bread crumbs. Using your hands, gently combine the mixture. Spoon into a 9 x 5-inch loaf pan. Flatten the top. Bake for 40 minutes, or until cooked through.

4. Meanwhile, cook the potatoes in boiling water to cover in a medium saucepan for 12 minutes, or until tender. Drain.

5. Return to an empty pan over low heat; stir to dry out the potatoes. Add the butter and milk and mash to the desired consistency. Season with salt and pepper.

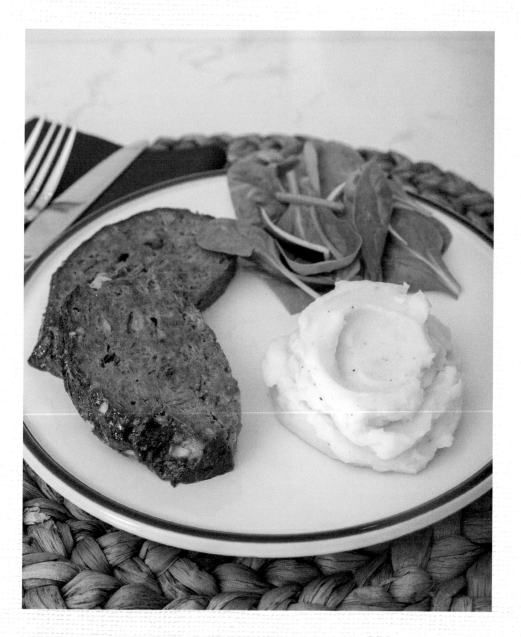

Day 2

Speedy Spaghetti with Meat Sauce

SERVES 4

EveryGirl
TIP: There are many tomato sauces available at the market that already have herbs or flavorings added, but I prefer to add my own veggies and herbs.

¾ pound spaghetti or other long pasta (regular, whole-wheat, or gluten-free)

1 tablespoon olive oil

1 medium onion, chopped

1 pound ground beef

1 teaspoon chopped garlic

Salt and black pepper

14 ounces tomato sauce

1 dried bay leaf

1. Cook the pasta according to the package directions. Drain.

2. Warm the oil in a medium saucepan over medium-low heat. Add the onion; cook, stirring, for 5 minutes, or until softened.

3. Add the beef and garlic, and salt and pepper to taste; cook for 8 minutes, stirring, until the beef is browned.

4. Add the sauce and bay leaf; cook for 8 minutes, stirring occasionally and adding water if the mixture seems too dry.

5. Remove the bay leaf. In a large serving bowl, toss the pasta with the hot sauce.

Day 3

Greek Lentil Salad with Lemon Dressing

SERVES 4

Lentil Salad
1 cup lentils
1 cup corn
2 cloves garlic, chopped
2 tablespoons dried parsley
2 tablespoons minced onion
Salt and black pepper

Dressing
¼ cup fresh lemon juice
¼ cup olive oil

EveryGirl
TIP: Lentils come in different colors and sizes. If you can find the tiny ones (called Le Puy or French lentils), use them. Otherwise, the traditional larger brown ones are fine.

1. In a medium saucepan over medium-high heat, combine the lentils, corn, garlic, and 2 cups of water. Bring to a boil, reduce the heat, and simmer for 25 minutes, or until just tender.

2. Stir in the parsley in the last two minutes of cooking time. Add more water if needed. Drain.

3. For the dressing: In a large serving bowl, whisk together the lemon juice and oil, until combined.

4. Add the lentils, minced onion, and season with salt and pepper to taste.

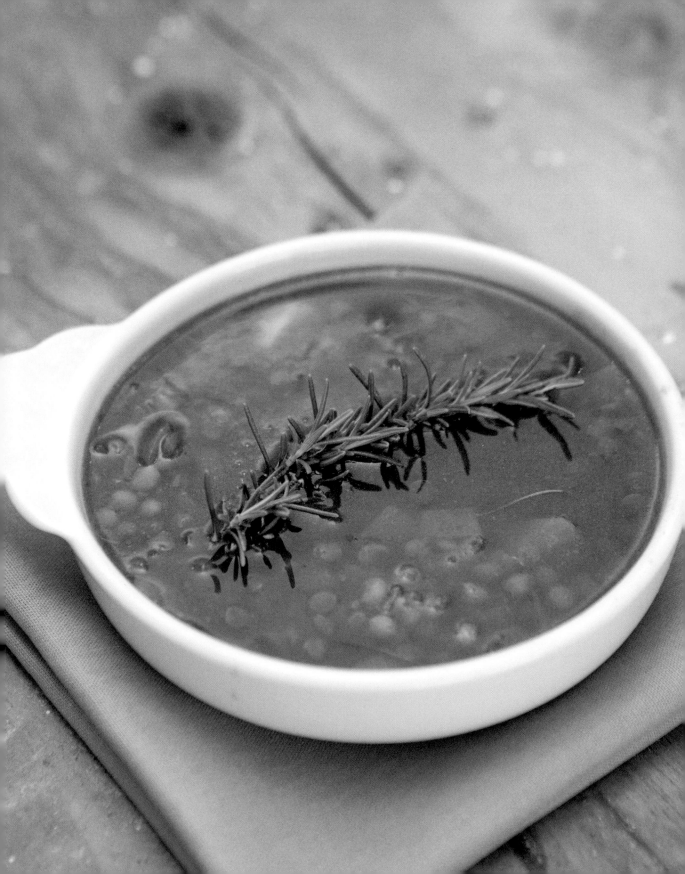

Day 4

Lentil Soup

SERVES 4

EveryGirl
TIP: Remove the bay leaves from the soup before serving.

½ pound lentils, rinsed

1 tablespoon diced onion

3 cloves garlic, chopped

2 dried bay leaves

1 teaspoon dried rosemary

¼ cup white or red wine vinegar, as desired

1 can (8 ounces) tomato sauce

¼ cup olive oil

Salt and pepper

1. In a medium saucepan, cook the lentils in water to cover for 25 minutes, or until just tender.

2. Add the onion, garlic, bay leaves, rosemary, vinegar, tomato sauce, and olive oil; cook for an additional 15 minutes, adding water if needed for the desired consistency.

3. Remove the bay leaf, season with salt and pepper to taste, and serve.

Day 5

Grilled Lemon Chicken with Creamed Spinach Mashed Potatoes

SERVES 4

¼ cup olive oil

1 tablespoon lemon juice

½ teaspoon dried oregano

Salt and black pepper

4 small boneless, skinless chicken breast halves

3 medium russet potatoes

4 tablespoons (½-stick) unsalted butter

1 box (6 ounces) fresh baby spinach

¾ cup low-fat milk, warmed

EveryGirl

TIP: Grilling times can vary greatly, and since boneless chicken breasts cook quickly, keep an eye on the grill.

EveryGirl

TIP: Russet potatoes, or Idaho potatoes, are the best choice for mashing, since they fall apart during the cooking process. Yukon Gold potatoes, or red potatoes, also called boiling potatoes, are best for salads, since they keep their shape.

1. In a large resealable plastic bag, combine the oil, lemon juice, oregano, and salt and pepper to taste. Add the chicken, seal the bag, and flip a few times to coat. Refrigerate for at least 4 hours or up to 12 hours.

2. Cook the potatoes in a large pot of boiling salted water for about 40 minutes, until tender. Drain and allow to cool. Peel the potatoes and coarsely chop.

3. Melt the butter in the same pot over medium-low heat. Add the spinach; cook for 2 minutes, or until wilted, stirring. Add the chopped potatoes and warm milk and mash with the spinach. Season with salt and pepper to taste.

4. Meanwhile, preheat the grill to high. Remove the chicken from the bag; discard the marinade. Grill the chicken until cooked through. Serve as individual portions by placing a mound of potatoes on the plate and nestle the chicken in the potatoes or transfer to serving bowls for the table.

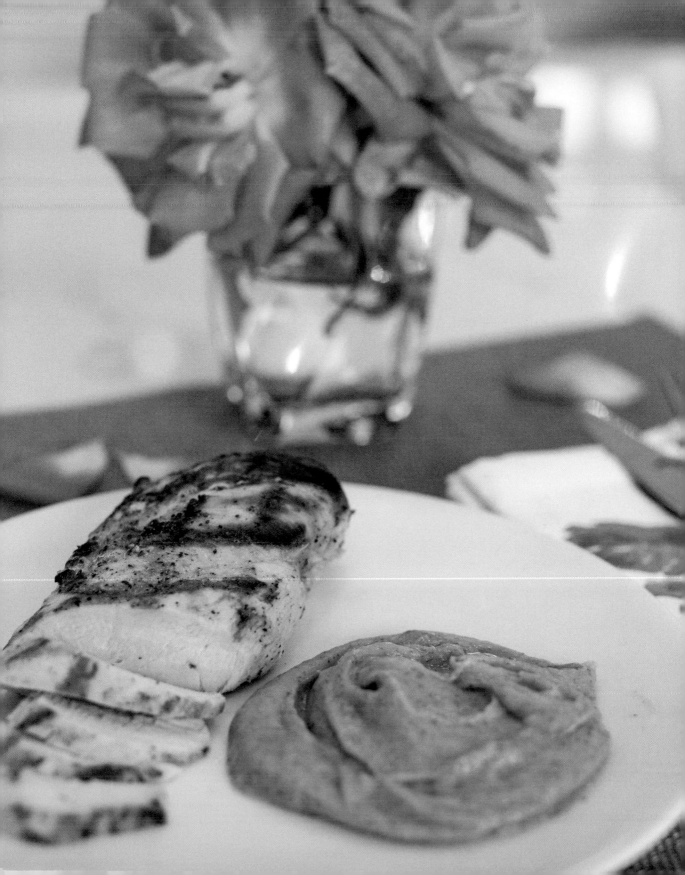

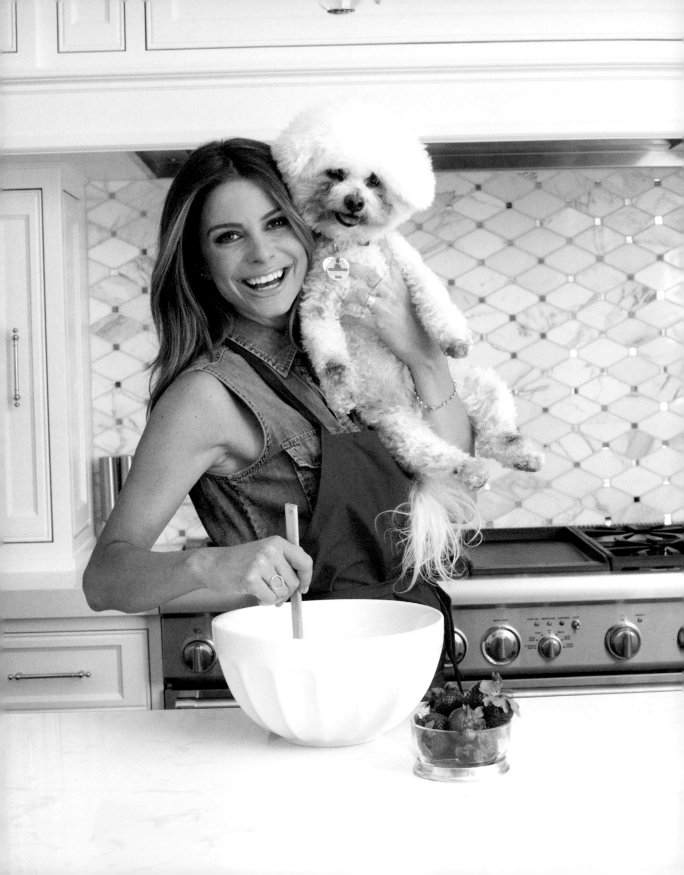

EveryGirl

COOKS FOR HER CANINE BABY

While shooting the cover for this book, I took some photos with Benjamin. I love the pictures and him so much that I wish I could have used them for the cover. Not sure how that would have looked on a cookbook for humans, but luckily I can use them in this special chapter.

Seeing the photos inspired me to help you guys with some everyday doggy problems. I enlisted the help of my friend and veterinarian, Dr. Brian Spar. Brian has helped me in the middle of the night on numerous occasions when I've been panicked over one of my sick pups. Many of the remedies are his suggestions from those actual moments! I also enlisted the help of two vet technicians, Erin Shaw and Natalie Ewing of DogVacay's Trust & Safety Team. These ladies spend their days answering the emails and phone calls of thousands of dog lovers who need advice about how to best care for the pups in their lives.

EveryPup

TIP: My doggy bible still to this day is *The Nature of Animal Healing* by Dr. Martin Goldstein. It's a great read and it has great holistic solutions for your dog.

EveryPup

TIP: Please avoid giving your dog peanut butter unless it is to get medicine down. Peanut butter is very high in fat and can lead to pancreatitis.

We have all been there. Our dog is sick and won't eat. Or hasn't gone #2 in days. Or has an upset tummy. Here are some recipes with the key ingredients that can help you with these and other issues, though you should always consult with your vet first, as your pup may have certain sensitivities or ailments I'm not aware of!

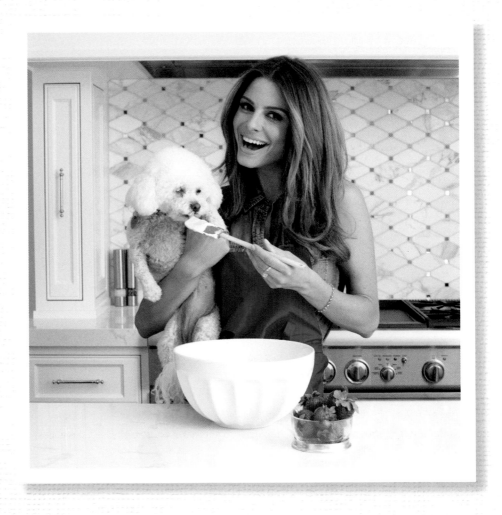

Canine Mini Patties

GOOD FOR: ALLERGIES   NOTE: KEEP REFRIGERATED.

1 pound salmon

2 large organic sweet potatoes

1 large egg

½ cup rolled oats

1. Preheat the oven to 400°F.

2. Boil the salmon in 2 cups water. When the fillets are cooked through, drain and let them cool. Once they're cool enough to touch, shred each one with a fork.

3. Bake the sweet potatoes at 400°F for 45 minutes. Mash the sweet potatoes together with the shredded salmon.

4. Beat the egg and add to the sweet potato and salmon mixture. Add the rolled oats to the mixture, and stir well.

5. Finally, make 1-inch patties (they can be a little larger, depending on your pup's size and appetite!) with the salmon mixture and bake at 350°F for 15 to 20 minutes.

6. Remove from the oven (you can break one patty open to make sure it's cooked all the way through) and let cool before serving to your pup.

Dr. Brian's Tip: This treat would hit all the areas of concern for allergic dogs—anti-inflammatory effects, increased skin barrier to allergens, palatability, and novel easy-to-find protein.

Erin/Natalie says: "These patties are great treats for dogs who have sensitivities to certain foods."

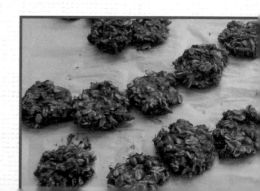

EveryPup Skinny Treat

GREAT FOR: EVERYPUP WHO IS OVERWEIGHT.

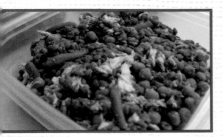

Benjamin has always been overweight. I even call him my little piggy. Oh, how I love my little chubby baby. But when things get out of control, I place him on a green bean diet. I know a lot of you like to give your dogs treats, so you can use this as a small treat or as a meal.

Dr. Brian's Tip: "The majority of my patients are overweight to some degree, usually because of all of the treats or table food their moms/dads feed them. Replacing junk food with treats like these (containing lean protein and fresh veggies) will help make your pet feel fuller with less caloric intake. It's a win-win!"

Erin/Natalie says: "If your pup has put on an extra pound or two, these are a great skinny treat to offer."

EveryPup

TIP: If your dog is overweight, split his normal meal portion in half and substitute one half with rinsed and drained canned green beans. This will help him lean out in no time. The beans are full of fiber and very filling.

10 cups water

1 whole organic chicken, cut into 8 pieces

1 pound uncooked lentils, rinsed

2 cups peas

2 cups green beans

1. Bring the water to a boil in a large pot over high heat. When the water is boiling, add the chicken. Boil for 15 minutes.

2. Add the lentils, peas, and beans, stir, and bring to a boil. Reduce the heat to medium-low and simmer for 30 minutes.

3. Let cool. Remove the skin and bones from the chicken. Drain the mixture if needed.

4. Freeze in individual serving-size plastic containers or resealable bags. Remember portions especially if serving as a treat. This should last awhile.

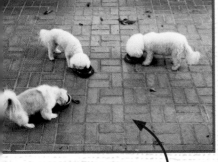

My babies loved this treat!

Pumpkin Bites

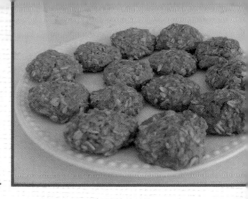

MAKES 40 QUARTER-SIZE BITES

GREAT FOR: EVERYPUP WHO IS CONSTIPATED OR HAS DIARRHEA.

NOTE: BE SURE TO KEEP REFRIGERATED.

Pumpkin is a great help in this department. Store a few cans of it on your pantry shelf for such an occasion. Here's a recipe your dog will surely love in its moment of need.

Dr. Brian's Tip: "Pumpkin is a wonderful natural source of fiber, which can help pups with either diarrhea or constipation. This, combined with a bland diet (like boiled skinless chicken breast and rice), is my initial go-to recommendation for my patients with intestinal distress. Most of the time, it helps tremendously without my having to prescribe any medications!"

Erin/Natalie says: "Pumpkin (or sweet potato) is your best friend when your pup is having tummy troubles! Whether his stools are loose or he's having the opposite issue, a little of this stuff will have him regular in no time."

> ½ cup Greek yogurt (make sure it's Greek yogurt, because it has the most protein)
> 1 cup canned 100% pure pumpkin puree
> 1¾ cups rolled oats

1. Preheat the oven to 350°F. Line a cookie sheet with parchment paper, and grease if necessary.

2. In a large bowl, stir together the yogurt and pumpkin. Stir in the oats, ¼ cup at a time, just until the dough is no longer sticky. Scoop the mixture out with a teaspoon or something small, and flatten into patties.

3. Bake at 350°F for 8 to 10 minutes. Let cool completely. Store in an airtight container or freeze for up to 3 months.

EveryPup
TIP: You can also give your dog pumpkin straight from the can if he's constipated. Dr. Brian advised me of that once and it worked like a charm!

EveryPup
TIP: Remember to keep your purses off the floor and out of reach of your dogs. I cannot tell you how many times I've seen dogs get into gum or candy, leading to thousands of dollars in vet bills!

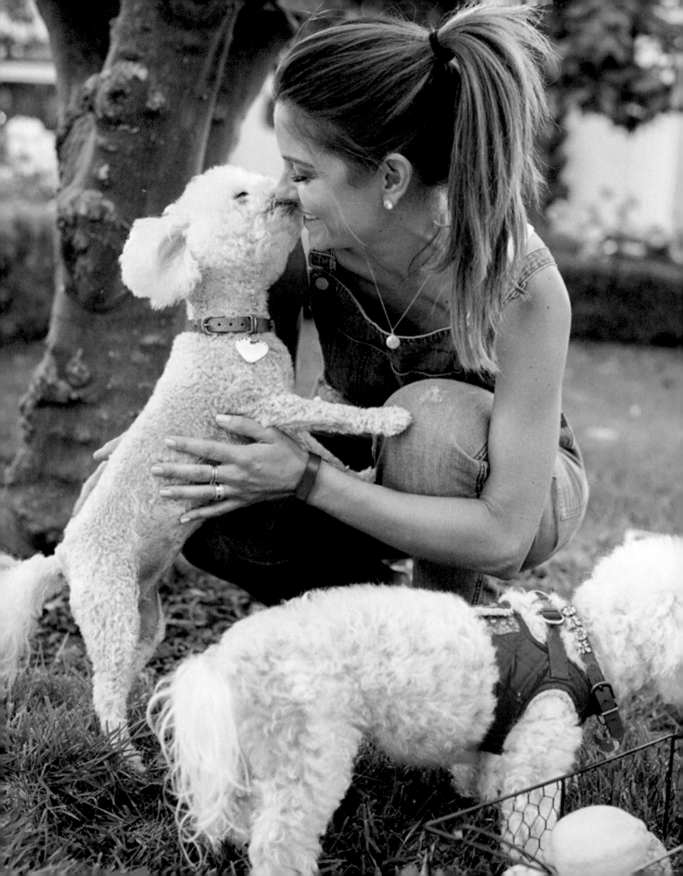

EveryGirl DOGGY COOKING MOMENT

If you know me, you know I view pets as bona fide members of the family. I currently have three . . . dogs: Baby, 15; Benjamin (Benny), 15; and Winnie, 4—and care very much about what I feed them. What they eat and what your dog eats will greatly affect their quality and length of life. What you serve up can also help common doggy ailments. When my babies get diarrhea, we feed them boiled rice. When they are constipated, we give them pumpkin. One time my girl, Baby, had bladder stones. The vet recommended surgery, which was both expensive and surely painful. Kev's mom suggested adding CranActin (a cranberry extract powder) to Baby's meals. In a few weeks, the stones had dissolved. It doesn't always work, but it did for us.

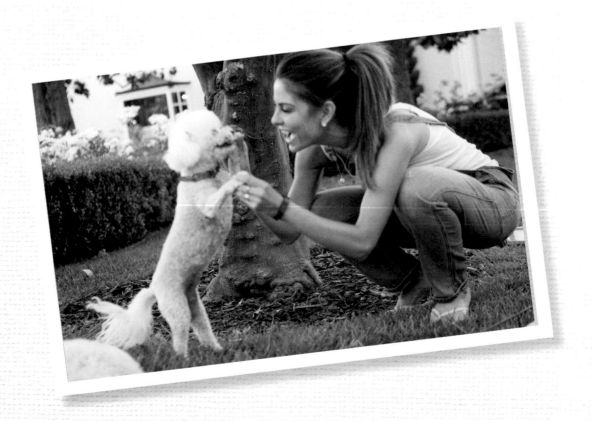

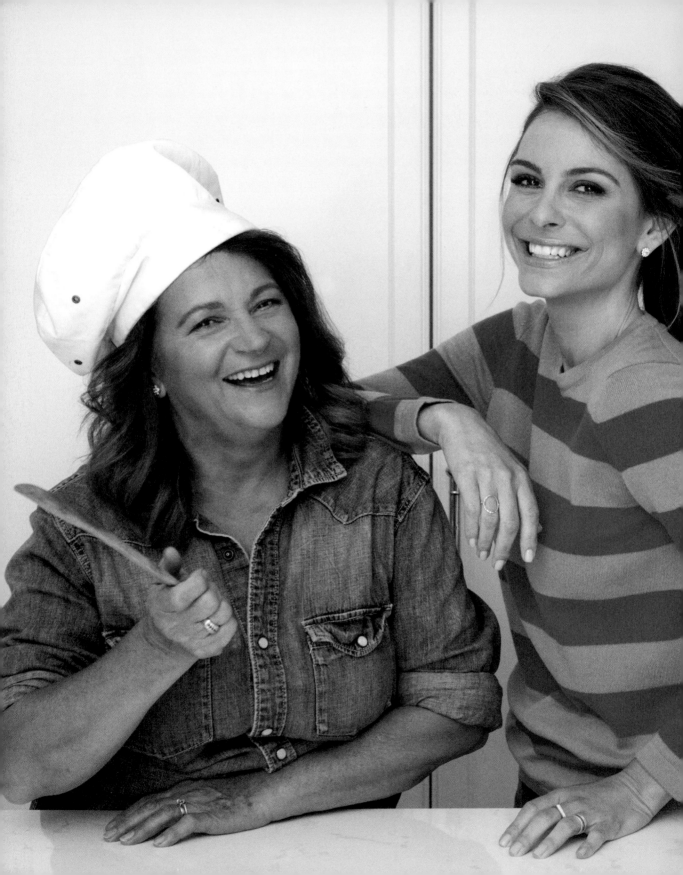

Kitchen

SIMPLE—BASIC KITCHEN TOOLS

I clearly remember the day I decided I was going to splurge and go to one of those fancy cookware stores. The plan was to outfit my newly remodeled kitchen with the "best" cookware on the market. At the time, I was still using cast-off pots that my mother had given me from our house in Medford, MA. Well, when I went to the store and looked at the new sets, I got overwhelmed. "Who needs all of this?" I thought. I've cooked for forty-plus people at my house during the holidays, and my mom's old pots and the few that I've added along the way work just fine. The lesson I learned was that you don't need to spend a fortune and buy a battery of equipment in order to cook delicious meals. You just need a few basic and multipurpose items made from sturdy materials that will last. Buy the best-quality cookware you can afford, but that doesn't necessarily mean buying the most expensive. Start with these bare-bones suggestions, then as you discover your own cooking style and passions, you can wisely add to your collection.

Serrated and regular chef's knives

Serrated knife

Paring knife

Sharpening steel

Knives: A chef knife is your most important tool. The best kind to buy has a stainless-steel, 8-inch blade. A serrated knife is perfect for slicing bread, tomatoes, and vegetables with tough skin. A paring knife is ideal for peeling. For all knives, help keep the blades sharp by washing your knives by hand, never in the dishwasher.

Two or three cast-aluminum saucepans (with lids): A 2-quart pot is useful for making sauces and cooking smaller batches of vegetables, pasta, and rice. A 4-quart pot works for soups, stews, and boiling water for pasta. If you like to make large batches of soup or pasta for a crowd, you'll also need a large (10- to 12-quart) stockpot. Whatever the size, you'll want one with a thick, heavy bottom to prevent burning. Thin pots will heat food unevenly.

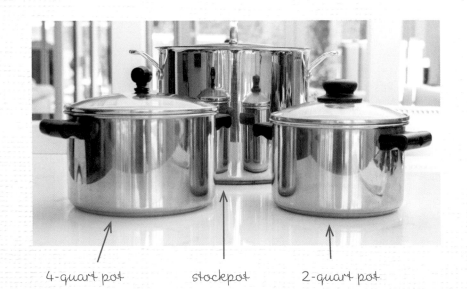

4-quart pot   stockpot   2-quart pot

Two skillets (with lids): An 8-inch nonstick skillet is perfect for fried eggs, omelets, and small dishes for one or two servings. You'll also need a 12-inch skillet that could hold two large steaks. This large skillet could be nonstick or cast iron. If you can afford it, buy one of each. Cast iron will last forever and is wonderful for cooking meats. A nonstick skillet is a good all-purpose choice for sautéing, frying, or stir-frying. Look for skillets with oven-safe handles, so the pan can go from the stovetop to the oven. Although easy to clean, the surface of nonstick skillets generally lasts for only a few years.

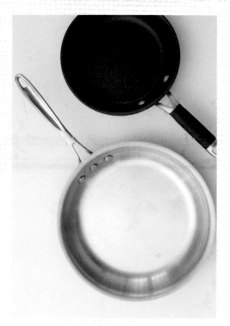

One sheet pan or baking sheet (not shown) is needed for baking cookies and pizzas, toasting nuts, and roasting vegetables. Get the largest one that will fit in your oven, preferably with a ½-inch rim.

One 9 x 13-inch baking pan for brownies, lasagna, and casseroles. If you like to bake quick breads, get a 9 x 5-inch loaf pan. For even baking, look for ones made from dark aluminum.

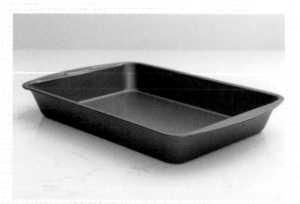
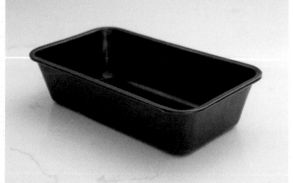

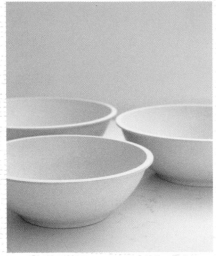

Stainless steel or plastic bowls are workhorses that you can use for just about any task.

A large colander with a base works for straining, draining, and rinsing pasta, beans, fruit, and vegetables. Stainless steel is preferable to plastic—although more expensive, it will last forever. Plastic easily stains and may melt if left on a hot stovetop.

It's a good idea to have two cutting boards (not shown), one for meats and one for everything else. Although wooden boards look better, plastic is lighter and can go in the dishwasher. Make sure they are large enough; a too-small cutting board hampers your work.

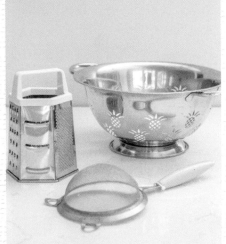

An upright grater is best for grating cheese, fruits, and vegetables. The three- or four-sided standing type is far easier to use than the flat type.

Sturdy tongs are the most underappreciated kitchen tool. Use them for grilling, to turn and grab fillets in a skillet, lifting hot lids off cooking pots, even stirring boiling pasta.

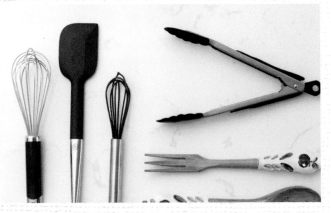

There are two different types of spatulas. A rubber spatula is great for stirring foods in nonstick skillets and mixing and scraping batters out of bowls. Make sure to buy one made of silicone or another heat-resistant material. A metal spatula is used to turn pancakes and remove cookies from baking sheets.

Wooden spoons are a must for cooking with nonstick skillets, since they won't scratch the surface. They are inexpensive, naturally beautiful, and will last forever (as long as you don't put them in the dishwasher!).

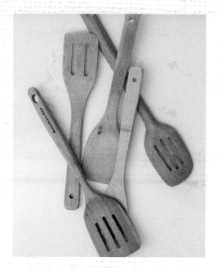

A slotted spoon has holes in it to drain any juices from meats you don't want to add to the plate.

If you bake a lot, get a **handheld or stand electric mixer**. Stand mixers are the gold standard for blending and beating batters and dough. However, they take up a lot of space in the kitchen and are quite pricey. Handheld mixers, although less powerful, are much cheaper and are well suited for most mixing jobs.

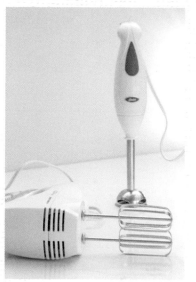

Food processors are great time-savers in the kitchen, but they are expensive. They make short work of big chopping and shredding jobs and can also do the work of a blender. I still love to use my Magic Bullet or buy pre-cut veggies when the budget allows!

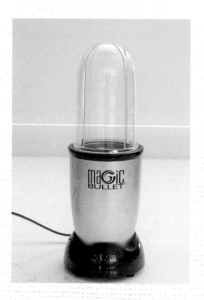

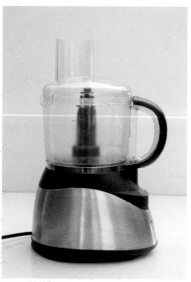

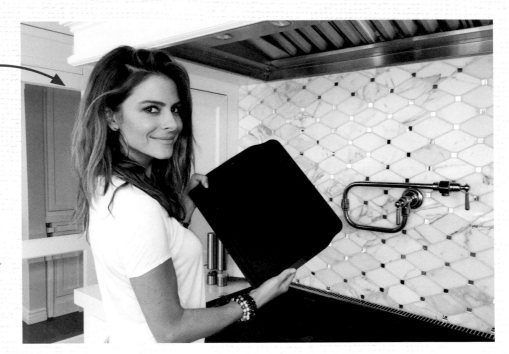

Like this backsplash? My friend Kelli has designed so many gorgeous pieces! Find them on Kelliellis.com

You might also want to get a **stovetop grill pan**—this fits over your stove burners and allows you to grill vegetables and meats inside (just make sure you have your stove's ventilation hood turned on!).

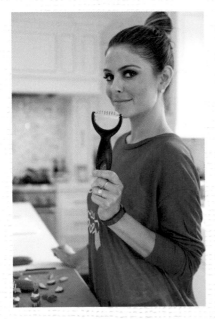

I also love my **vegetable peeler**. In addition to doing what its name says it should (peel vegetables), it's also a handy tool for creating ribbons of hard cheese like Parmesan.

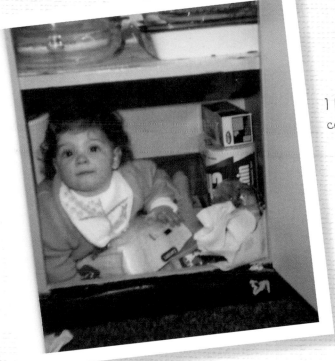

I liked hiding in cabinets!

EveryGirl COOKING MOMENT

You want to know *just* how much I love cooking and working in the kitchen? My mom recently reminded me that one time when I was little and she was cooking, I started doing the dishes. I didn't know what I was doing. I just wanted to be in the kitchen with her. I kept pouring soap out of the bottle and onto my hands and running them under hot water. Unfortunately, I took things a little too far—my hands got so irritated and chapped that I had to go to the doctor!

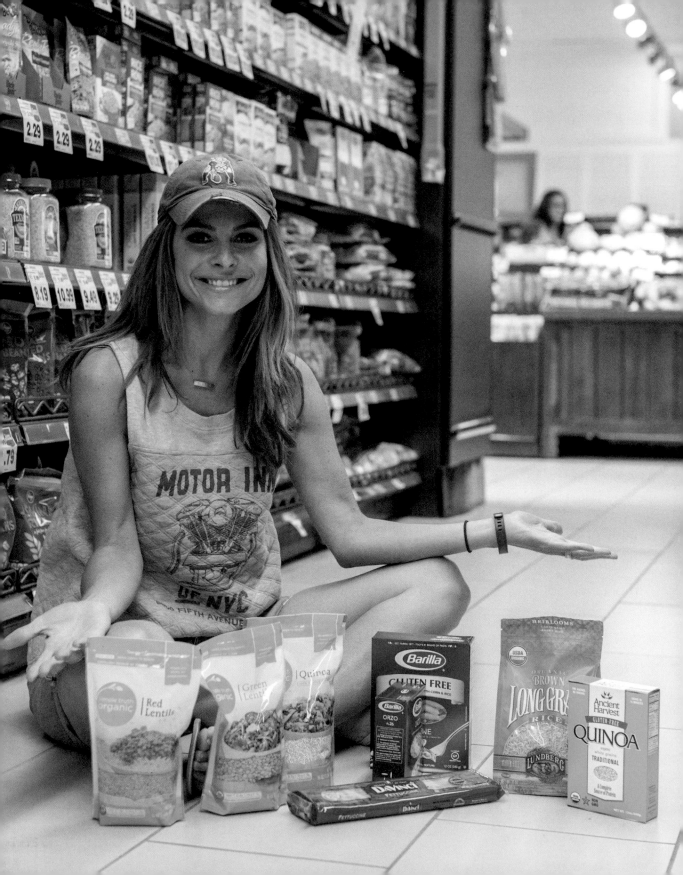

EveryGirl

PANTRY BASICS— ESSENTIAL INGREDIENTS

Sometimes reading a recipe ingredient list can be daunting for beginning cooks. You know that making a shopping list is your first step, but what if you are unclear about the ingredients you are supposed to buy? Here's some basic information about many of my pantry must-haves to make your next trip to the supermarket a breeze. If you really want to start cooking at home and want to use this book more than occasionally, I suggest stocking your pantry with them.

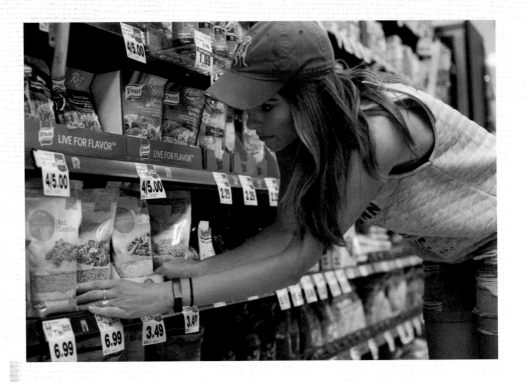

EveryGirl

TIP: Check out your local Dollar Store for cheap dried herbs and spices, and any kitchen items. Also Tuesday Morning has cookware at good prices.

Olive oil

Salt

Pepper

Granulated onion

Granulated garlic

Oregano

Dried mint

Dried anise

Dried parsley

Dried basil

Crushed red pepper

Flour

Tomato sauce

Chicken broth

Dried bay leaf

Dried rosemary

Lemon juice

Lime juice

Grated Parmesan cheese

Italian spices

Pasta

Spaghetti

Bread crumbs

Vinegar

Brown rice

Black beans

Garbanzo beans (chickpeas)

Kidney beans

Low-sodium green beans

White beans

Quinoa

• Oils and Fats

Olive oil is your best bet for cooking and salad dressings. Use the more-expensive extra-virgin olive oil for salad dressings and other uncooked dishes, so that its pure, fruity flavor can shine through. Pure olive oil (usually just called olive oil) is lighter in color and a bit blander, but is a great go-to oil for cooking. Light olive oil is even blander and not recommended.

Canola and vegetable oils can be used for frying, sautéing, and some baked goods. They lack the pure, non-greasy flavor of olive oil, so are not a good choice for salads.

Nonstick cooking spray can be used for greasing, cooking, and baking pans. Although it doesn't deliver the flavor of olive oil, it can be a low-fat technique. Just remember if you are greasing your skillet with cooking spray rather than oil, foods tend to burn more quickly, so you may need to reduce the heat under the pan.

Butter imparts a delicious rich flavor to dishes. Since it is a less-healthy fat option, it is best used in small amounts to finish sauces, or in baking special treats. Store butter in the freezer if you use it infrequently.

• Salt and Pepper

Table salt is fine-grained and contains additives to make it flow freely. Kosher salt is a coarse-grained, additive-free salt that delivers better flavor than table salt. Both types can be used in both sweet and savory dishes. Sea salt is made from the evaporation of seawater. It has the best flavor of all salts, but is very expensive. Save it for a finishing salt—to sprinkle on, to taste, just before serving.

Black pepper is available either ground or as whole peppercorns. Although I prefer freshly ground pepper for its stronger flavor, you will need to invest in a pepper mill to grind the corns. Jars of ground pepper are inexpensive, but lose their flavor within a few months. Whole peppercorns will keep for at least a year.

Cayenne pepper is actually a ground mixture of dried chili peppers. It will add a spicy kick to a dish. Crushed red pepper (or red pepper flakes) is also a mixture of dried chili peppers, but contains the crushed seeds and pods of the pepper. In either case, a little bit goes a long way, so add it sparingly unless you want a lot of heat.

• Herbs

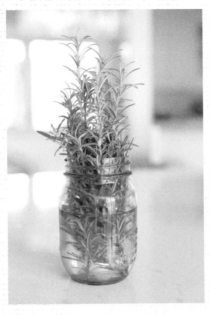
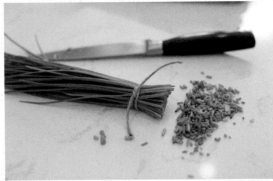

For some recipes, like uncooked salads, it's best to use fresh herbs. To prep, strip the leaves from the stem and, using a sharp knife, chop the leaves into small pieces. For long-cooking soups or roasted meats, you can use fresh or dried herbs. However, dried herbs are stronger in flavor, so my general rule is to use about half as much dried herbs as fresh herbs.

Dried herbs should be stored, tightly sealed, in a cool place out of direct sunlight. Using a marker, write the purchase date on the jar. They will last from one to three years. Fresh herbs will last a week if stored correctly. Soft herbs, like parsley, cilantro, and tarragon, should be stored like a bouquet of flowers, in a glass of water, and be kept in the refrigerator. Loosely cover the top with a plastic bag. Hard herbs, like rosemary and thyme, should be stored in plastic bags in the crisper of your refrigerator. For all fresh herbs, don't wash them until just before chopping and adding to a dish.

• Spices

Spices are available in either whole or ground form. The majority of recipes (mine and others') call for ground spices, so unless you have a spice grinder, buy pre-ground. Unless you know you will be using a spice often, buy the smallest jar you can find. Store, tightly sealed, in a cool, dark place, out of direct sunlight. Using a marker, write the purchase date on the jar, so you can keep track of its freshness, but know that spices will last from two to three years.

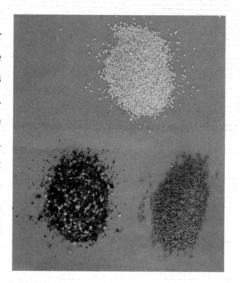

• Rice and Grains

All types of grains are good sources of complex carbohydrates and are low in fat. Your best bet are those labeled as whole grains, which haven't undergone the process to remove their germ and bran. These unrefined grains are higher in fiber and other essential nutrients.

There are many gluten-free whole-grain options on the market these days, such as brown rice, wild rice, quinoa, and millet. Although most of these grains can be used interchangeably in recipes, each has its own cooking method, so check the package directions before cooking.

Save money and reduce waste by buying grains in bulk when possible. To maintain freshness and reduce spoilage, store grains tightly sealed in a cool, dark place.

• Pasta

The pasta shelves are increasingly packed with options—no longer just regular and whole-grain. There are even gluten-free varieties, including rice, corn, and quinoa pasta. Although you can swap them out for regular pasta in recipes, cooking times vary, so check the package directions. If you have gluten sensitivity, try out some of the options to see which you like best.

• Vinegars

Vinegar adds a bright, acidic taste to salads, sauces, and marinades. For best flavor, add vinegar to a cooked dish *after* it is removed from the heat.

Apple-cider vinegar has a tart, fruity flavor. It is inexpensive and widely available. Red- and white-wine vinegars are made from fermented wine and work especially well in salad dressings and cooked vegetable dishes. Balsamic vinegar is made from a grape variety. It adds a complex tart-sweet flavor to dishes, but can be very expensive.

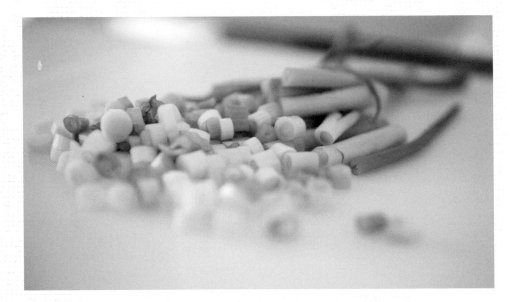

• Onions and Garlic

Some of the most delicious recipes start with the simplest ingredients: onions and garlic. These two humble foods provide a flavorful base from which a wide variety of recipes begin. Both are available year-round and will keep for a couple of months if stored in a cool, dry place with good air circulation. Do not refrigerate.

Onions add a sweet, earthy flavor when sautéed and a spicy punch when used fresh. Use yellow and red onions for long-cooking dishes. Reach for milder scallions and shallots for salads and uncooked dishes.

Garlic is sold by the head—each head made up of several individual cloves and wrapped in its own papery skin. Break off the number of cloves needed and peel off the skin before mincing the clove with a sharp knife.

• Tomatoes and Tomato Sauces

Canned tomatoes and tomato sauce are essential pantry staples for soups, stews, and other cooked dishes. They are inexpensive, convenient, and ready to use, since the tomatoes are already peeled, seeded, and chopped. Both products also contain lycopene, a carotenoid that has been found to prevent prostate and breast cancer.

Fresh tomatoes are delicious in August, but offer a mealy mouthful in January. Celebrate their season and use them in salads and uncooked dishes, during late summer and early fall. Cherry tomatoes are your best fresh-taste choice during the winter and spring months. For best flavor and texture, never refrigerate fresh tomatoes, unless they've been cut.

• Beans

Most beans are available both dried and canned. They can be used interchangeably in recipes and deliver the same (stellar) nutritional benefits. However, dried beans need to be cooked before using, and canned beans are ready to eat.

Dried beans are cheap and environmentally friendly, using less packaging than canned beans. They are perfectly pure and natural—no additives. They will keep for years in a dark, dry storage space. The only downside is the cooking factor. Dried beans can take an hour or more to cook. Many varieties need to be soaked overnight in advance of cooking, as well.

Canned beans are more expensive than dried, although still not costly. They are fast and convenient, as they are fully cooked. Just drain, rinse, and add to your dish. The downside? Canned beans sometimes contain preservatives and high levels of sodium. Check the ingredient label when choosing your brand.

• Canned Fish

Canned fish, like tuna, salmon, and crabmeat, is an affordable protein source that will keep in your pantry for months. Although canned fish doesn't deliver the same flavor as a fresh fillet, it is great to have on hand for salads and sandwiches. Reduce added fat by selecting fish packed in water rather than oil. Since canned fish is higher in sodium than fresh fish, read the label before buying.

• Broth

Broth is a liquid flavored with meat scraps or vegetables and is used as a flavor base for soups, stews, and other cooked dishes. You'll find it in the soup aisle of your market and is sometimes called "stock." Swap out broth for water when making rice or soups to enhance flavor.

Buy broth labeled "reduced-sodium," so that you can control the amount of salt in your dish.

• Cheese

It's always best to buy a block of cheese and grate or crumble it yourself. Although the pre-shredded varieties save time, they are more expensive. These processed cheeses also often contain additives that have nothing to do with cheese. More important, the flavor of block cheese is infinitely better than the pre-shredded.

There are many types of feta cheese in the markets. For freshest flavor, buy feta blocks that are packaged in brine. You might have to travel to a specialty cheese shop, but it's worth it!

• Citrus Fruits

Always use fresh lemons and limes when a recipe calls for juice. Bottled juice, although convenient, tastes unnatural and often contains additives. To have juice always on hand, buy lemons and limes when on sale and squeeze the juice into ice cube trays. Once frozen, put the cubes into resealable plastic bags and freeze for up to six months. You could even grow a small tree in a pot; you don't need a large space and will still receive tons of fruit.

Lemon and lime zest is the colored part of the skin. It's sometimes referred to as the peel, but technically, the peel is the entire outer shell, including the bitter white part. No matter what it's called, use only the colored zest, using the fine holes of a grater to remove.

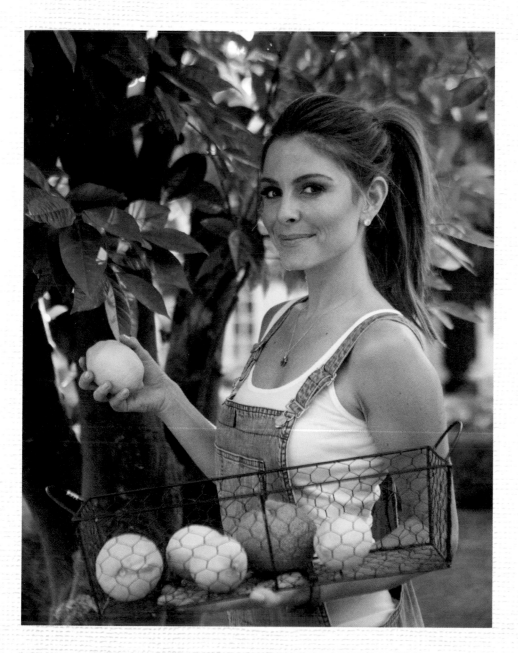

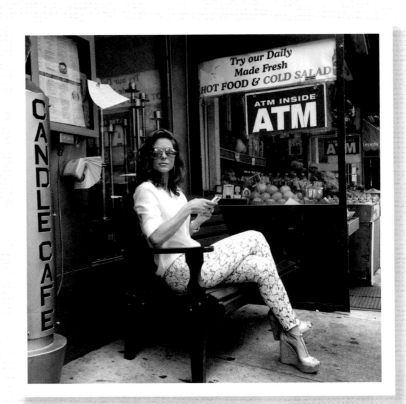

Final Words

I hope this book helps you get past any cooking insecurities and teaches you how to cook delicious, healthy recipes. I also hope you will tag me on social media as you make these recipes and entertain. I really love interacting with all of you and learning from you, too! And remember:

Anything is possible. You can do anything you put your mind to. Think out of the box. Reach for the stars, and work hard on your peer group. And don't forget to dream!

everygirl.com

conversationswithmaria.com

theeverygirlsguide@gmail.com

Twitter & Instagram: @mariamenounos #EveryGirlCooking

A Note from the Doctors

We all need a dose of healthy carbohydrates for our body every day. In fact, our brain relies on carbs as its fuel source. When thinking about carbohydrates, we need to think about what healthy carbs are and which ones give us longer energy and keep us satisfied and full. Those are high-fiber carbs; high-fiber carbs (such as brown rice, quinoa, barley, sweet potatoes with skin, lentils, black beans, pinto beans, etc.) not only give a powerful energy punch but also keep our blood sugars more steady over a longer period of time. Soluble fibers found in a wide variety of whole organic grains, fruits, and vegetables slow the breakdown of carbohydrates in our body, thus releasing sugar into the bloodstream more slowly and steadily. Insoluble fibers found in many dark leafy vegetables, green beans, celery, and carrots help with providing regular bowel movements and healthy bowel function. Fibers also help with heart health, lowering cholesterol, and with weight management.

We have reviewed the recipes in this book and marked many that can be part of a healthful, carbohydrate-controlled diet. We recommend that our patients with type 2 diabetes Mellitus adhere to a consistent carbohydrate-controlled diet to help maintain stable blood sugar. Patients with type 2 diabetes have altered metabolism of blood glucose. Either their bodies have become resistant to the effects of insulin (the hormone that regulates the movement of sugar into cells), their bodies are no longer able to produce enough insulin to maintain normal blood glucose levels, or a combination of the two. (Patients with type 1 diabetes Mellitus lack the ability to produce any insulin from the pancreas.)

If you have questions about creating a meal plan recommended specifically for you, it is a good idea to meet with a registered dietitian to help you formulate concrete goals. Here are a few loose, general guidelines to follow to make a recipe diabetes-friendly.

Concentrate on those recipes that include higher amounts of vegetables and lower amounts of simple carbs (such as honey, agave, brown sugar, fruits, etc.) and also recipes containing lean proteins (like a minimum of 20 grams of protein per serving of entree).

Choose something that is fiber-rich (for example, 5 grams of fiber or more).

Please keep in mind what other sources of carbohydrate are in your meals in an effort not to exceed recommendations for each meal. Consider 30 grams of carbohydrates at breakfast and 45 to 60 grams of carbohydrates at lunch and dinner.

—Dr. Stephanie Smooke, endocrinology specialist, UCLA, and Sherly Cherian, RD, MPH, dietitian, Gonda Diabetes Center, UCLA

Acknowledgments

As with all books we've written, it truly takes a village. Allow me to take this moment to thank that village. Of course, I have to thank you, Mom, for all your work creating these recipes, and for loving me after the arguments that ensued! Keven, you are my partner in everything; thank you for all you do to help make these books come to life. No matter how much we have going on, how tired you are, you always make the time to make them amazing. Thank you for helping me create a series I am proud of, that helps other girls like me to live better lives. Dad, thanks for holding down the fort and taking care of the dogs while we were all busy writing and cooking!

A special thank-you to the Tsariannis family. You risked so much to help us in our time of need. I will forever be grateful.

I would also like to thank David Zinczenko, Marnie Cochran, Joe Perez, and the team at Galvanized and Random House. Marnie, thank you for all your guidance and incredible support in bringing this book to life. Susan Ott, you were a dream to work with. Thank you for all your hard work and patience! Thank you to Andy McNichol, for always helping me achieve my vision, Jon Rosen, Rich Gambale, Kevin Yorn, Nick Gladden, Ryan Goodell, and to the rest of my team at WME and Morris Yorn Barnes Levine et al. With all the projects I have going on, I know how hard it sometimes is for you. Thank you for your patience and devotion. To Gary Mantoosh and Brett Ruttenberg, likewise, your tireless efforts in the realm of publicity are incredible. I cannot thank you enough for your countless hours of work to get the Every-Girl's guides out there! Thank you. I would also like to thank Lois Wecker, Juliet Martin, and the team at Gelfand, Rennert & Feldman for all they do for me, as well as Glenn Rotner and Stacey Diament. Thank you, McKenzie, for helping transcribe Mom's recipes.

A special thank-you to Dr. Stephanie Smooke, endocrinology specialist, UCLA, and Sherly Cherian, RD, MPH, dietitian, Gonda Diabetes Center, UCLA, for all their help identifying the recipes key for diabetics and gluten-free individuals.

To my EveryGirl team, we prepped, cooked, photographed, and ate these delicious dishes that now burst off the pages of this book. Thank you, Mom, Elise, Marci, Violeta, Signa, Susan, and Tammie for your passion, love, and determination. Elise Donoghue, our collaboration on the photos for all of my books has been a dream. You are so talented, passionate, fast, and fun. I couldn't dream of doing this without you. Signa Brus, your dedication to this book has been beyond my wildest dreams. I'm so lucky to have you in my corner and so thankful for everything you did to help me see this to fruition. Dimitri Giannetos, my love, you have changed my life. Thank you for always making me feel and look my best and for teaching me so much. I love you so much. And thank you for the chef's hat idea for the cover—so fun!

To my EveryGirls out there who have been on this journey with me from the first book, I love you all. Thank you for supporting me and for spreading the word about these books. I will always do right by all of you.

Index

About the Authors

MARIA MENOUNOS is co-anchor and managing editor of *E! News,* an actress, and the two-time *New York Times* bestselling author of her EveryGirl's Guide book series: *The EveryGirl's Guide to Life* and *The EveryGirl's Guide to Diet and Fitness.* As host of the National CineMedia's *First Look Cinema Pre-Show,* she is seen daily, seven days a week, on 70 percent of America's movie screens. At SiriusXM, Maria hosts a daily afternoon drive series, "Conversations with Maria Menounos," interviewing celebrities and influencers. At twenty-two, she was, and remains, the youngest person to host *Entertainment Tonight.* Reporting for NBC's *Nightly News,* she is also the only journalist to interview the entire Obama family. A semifinalist on *Dancing with the Stars,* Menounos is also a part-time wrestler for the WWE, and is the creator and executive producer of ABC's *#DanceBattle America* alongside Keven Undergaro and Julianne Hough. In addition, Menounos co-founded AfterBuzz TV with partner, Keven Undergaro: an online broadcast network dedicated to producing after-shows for your favorite TV shows. The network is the largest of its kind, playing to more than 20+ million weekly in more than 100 countries. She recently created and launched her own Greek food line with her mother, Maria's Greek Delights.

KEVEN UNDERGARO is a TV producer, filmmaker, entrepreneur, brand builder, and co-author of *The EveryGirl's Guide to Life* and *The EveryGirl's Guide to Diet and Fitness* with longtime partner, Maria Menounos. Undergaro is the creator of the world's largest online broadcast network, AfterBuzz TV, and the first urban network, Black Hollywood Live, as well as the Popcorn Talk Network and Book Circle Online, for movie and book discussion respectively. His networks produce more than 100 shows weekly and have a roster of more than 200 hosts.